Antimicrobial Use across Different Healthcare Settings, Countries and Specific Populations

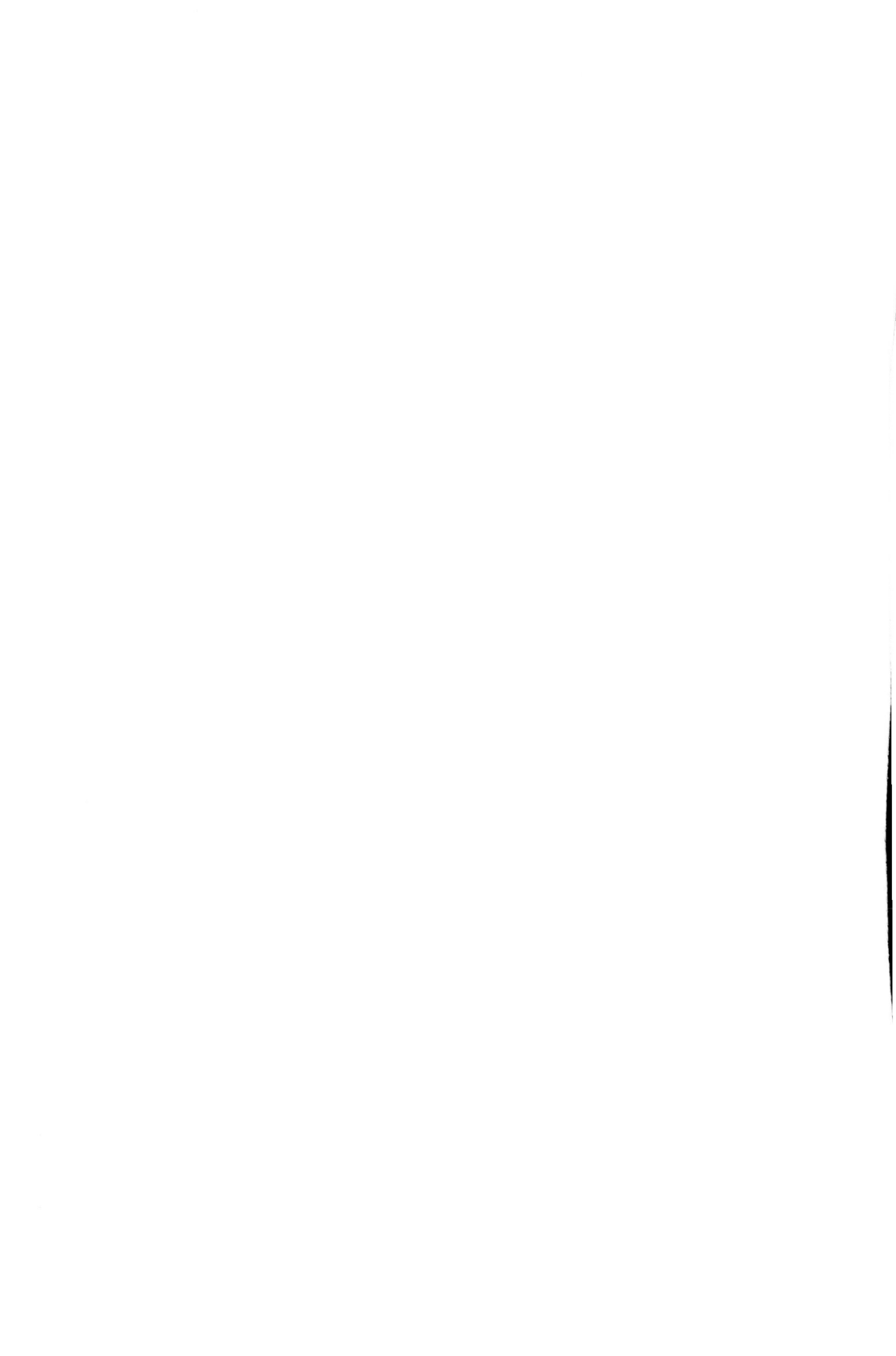

Antimicrobial Use across Different Healthcare Settings, Countries and Specific Populations

Editors

Gyöngyvér Soós
Ria Benkő

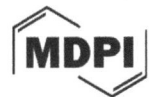 Basel • Beijing • Wuhan • Barcelona • Belgrade • Novi Sad • Cluj • Manchester

Gyöngyvér Soós
Department of
Clinical Pharmacy
University of Szeged
Szeged
Hungary

Ria Benkő
Department of
Clinical Pharmacy
University of Szeged
Szeged
Hungary

Editorial Office
MDPI AG
Grosspeteranlage 5
4052 Basel, Switzerland

This is a reprint of articles from the Special Issue published online in the open access journal *Antibiotics* (ISSN 2079-6382) (available at: www.mdpi.com/journal/antibiotics/special_issues/Healthcare_Settings).

For citation purposes, cite each article independently as indicated on the article page online and using the guide below:

Lastname, A.A.; Lastname, B.B. Article Title. *Journal Name* **Year**, *Volume Number*, Page Range

ISBN 978-3-7258-1534-0 (Hbk)
ISBN 978-3-7258-1533-3 (PDF)
https://doi.org/10.3390/books978-3-7258-1533-3

© 2024 by the authors. Articles in this book are Open Access and distributed under the Creative Commons Attribution (CC BY) license. The book as a whole is distributed by MDPI under the terms and conditions of the Creative Commons Attribution-NonCommercial-NoDerivs (CC BY-NC-ND) license (https://creativecommons.org/licenses/by-nc-nd/4.0/).

Contents

Gaetano Iaquinto, Giuseppe Mazzarella, Carmine Sellitto, Angela Lucariello, Raffaele Melina and Salvatore Iaquinto et al.
Antibiotic Therapy for Active Crohn's Disease Targeting Pathogens: An Overview and Update
Reprinted from: *Antibiotics* 2024, 13, 151, doi:10.3390/antibiotics13020151 1

Carmen Hidalgo-Tenorio, Inés Pitto-Robles, Daniel Arnés García, F. Javier Membrillo de Novales, Laura Morata and Raul Mendez et al.
Cefto Real-Life Study: Real-World Data on the Use of Ceftobiprole in a Multicenter Spanish Cohort
Reprinted from: *Antibiotics* 2023, 12, 1218, doi:10.3390/antibiotics12071218 14

Marcella Sibani, Lorenzo Maria Canziani, Chiara Tonolli, Maddalena Armellini, Elena Carrara and Fulvia Mazzaferri et al.
Antimicrobial Stewardship in COVID-19 Patients: Those Who Sow Will Reap Even through Hard Times
Reprinted from: *Antibiotics* 2023, 12, 1009, doi:10.3390/antibiotics12061009 30

Loni Schramm, Mitchell K. Byrne and Taylor Sweetnam
Antibiotic Misuse Behaviours of Older People: Confirmation of the Factor Structure of the Antibiotic Use Questionnaire
Reprinted from: *Antibiotics* 2023, 12, 718, doi:10.3390/antibiotics12040718 42

Juliane Hauschild, Nora Bruns, Elke Lainka and Christian Dohna-Schwake
A European International Multicentre Survey on the Current Practice of Perioperative Antibiotic Prophylaxis for Paediatric Liver Transplantations
Reprinted from: *Antibiotics* 2023, 12, 292, doi:10.3390/antibiotics12020292 56

Maarten Lambert, Ria Benkő, Athina Chalkidou, Jesper Lykkegaard, Malene Plejdrup Hansen and Carl Llor et al.
Developing a Tool for Auditing the Quality of Antibiotic Dispensing in Community Pharmacies: A Pilot Study
Reprinted from: *Antibiotics* 2022, 11, 1529, doi:10.3390/antibiotics11111529 66

Manas K. Akmatov, Claudia Kohring, Lotte Dammertz, Joachim Heuer, Maike Below and Jörg Bätzing et al.
The Effect of the COVID-19 Pandemic on Outpatient Antibiotic Prescription Rates in Children and Adolescents—A Claims-Based Study in Germany
Reprinted from: *Antibiotics* 2022, 11, 1433, doi:10.3390/antibiotics11101433 81

Peter Konstantin Kurotschka, Chiara Fulgenzio, Roberto Da Cas, Giuseppe Traversa, Gianluigi Ferrante and Orietta Massidda et al.
Effect of Fluoroquinolone Use in Primary Care on the Development and Gradual Decay of *Escherichia coli* Resistance to Fluoroquinolones: A Matched Case-Control Study
Reprinted from: *Antibiotics* 2022, 11, 822, doi:10.3390/antibiotics11060822 88

Anita Shallal, Chloe Lahoud, Dunia Merhej, Sandra Youssef, Jelena Verkler and Linda Kaljee et al.
The Impact of a Post-Prescription Review and Feedback Antimicrobial Stewardship Program in Lebanon
Reprinted from: *Antibiotics* 2022, 11, 642, doi:10.3390/antibiotics11050642 99

Adina Fésüs, Ria Benkő, Mária Matuz, Zsófia Engi, Roxána Ruzsa and Helga Hambalek et al.
Impact of Guideline Adherence on Outcomes in Patients Hospitalized with Community-Acquired Pneumonia (CAP) in Hungary: A Retrospective Observational Study
Reprinted from: *Antibiotics* **2022**, *11*, 468, doi:10.3390/antibiotics11040468 . . . . **109**

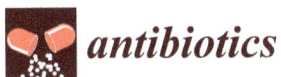

Review

Antibiotic Therapy for Active Crohn's Disease Targeting Pathogens: An Overview and Update

Gaetano Iaquinto [1], Giuseppe Mazzarella [2,3], Carmine Sellitto [4,5,*], Angela Lucariello [6], Raffaele Melina [7], Salvatore Iaquinto [8], Antonio De Luca [4] and Vera Rotondi Aufiero [2,3]

1. Gastroenterology Unit, St. Rita Hospital, 83042 Atripalda, Italy; iaquintog@yahoo.it
2. Institute of Food Sciences, Consiglio Nazionale Delle Ricerche (CNR), 83100 Atripalda, Italy; gmazzarella@isa.cnr.it (G.M.); vera.rotondiaufiero@isa.cnr.it (V.R.A.)
3. E.L.F.I.D, Department of Translational Medical Science, University "Federico II", 80147 Napoli, Italy
4. Section of Human Anatomy, Department of Mental and Physical Health and Preventive Medicine, University of Campania "Luigi Vanvitelli", 80138 Naples, Italy; antonio.deluca@unicampania.it
5. Department of Medicine, Surgery and Dentistry "Scuola Medica Salernitana", University of Salerno, 84081 Salerno, Italy
6. Department of Sport Sciences and Wellness, University of Naples "Parthenope", 80100 Naples, Italy; angela.lucariello@uniparthenope.it
7. Gastroenterology Unit, San G. Moscati Hospital, 83100 Atripalda, Italy; raffaelemelina@icloud.com
8. Gastroenterology Unit, St. Filippo Neri Hospital, 00135 Rome, Italy; salvatoreiaquinto@gmail.com
* Correspondence: csellitto@unisa.it; Tel.: +39-3491420236

Abstract: Crohn's disease (CD) is a multifactorial chronic disorder that involves a combination of factors, including genetics, immune response, and gut microbiota. Therapy includes salicylates, immunosuppressive agents, corticosteroids, and biologic drugs. International guidelines do not recommend the use of antibiotics for CD patients, except in the case of septic complications. Increasing evidence of the involvement of gut bacteria in this chronic disease supports the rationale for using antibiotics as the primary treatment for active CD. In recent decades, several pathogens have been reported to be involved in the development of CD, but only *Escherichia coli* (*E. coli*) and *Mycobacterium avium paratubercolosis* (MAP) have aroused interest due to their strong association with CD pathogenesis. Several meta-analyses have been published concerning antibiotic treatment for CD patients, but randomized trials testing antibiotic treatment against *E. coli* and MAP have not shown prolonged benefits and have generated conflicting results; several questions are still unresolved regarding trial design, antibiotic dosing, the formulation used, the treatment course, and the outcome measures. In this paper, we provide an overview and update of the trials testing antibiotic treatment for active CD patients, taking into account the role of pathogens, the mechanisms by which different antibiotics act on harmful pathogens, and antibiotic resistance. Finally, we also present new lines of study for the future regarding the use of antibiotics to treat patients with active CD.

Keywords: Crohn's disease; *Escherichia coli*; *Mycobacterium avium paratuberculosis*; antibiotic therapy

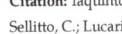

Citation: Iaquinto, G.; Mazzarella, G.; Sellitto, C.; Lucariello, A.; Melina, R.; Iaquinto, S.; De Luca, A.; Rotondi Aufiero, V. Antibiotic Therapy for Active Crohn's Disease Targeting Pathogens: An Overview and Update. *Antibiotics* **2024**, *13*, 151. https://doi.org/10.3390/antibiotics13020151

Academic Editors: Gyöngyvér Soós and Ria Benkő

Received: 5 January 2024
Revised: 29 January 2024
Accepted: 2 February 2024
Published: 3 February 2024

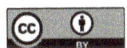

Copyright: © 2024 by the authors. Licensee MDPI, Basel, Switzerland. This article is an open access article distributed under the terms and conditions of the Creative Commons Attribution (CC BY) license (https://creativecommons.org/licenses/by/4.0/).

1. Introduction

Current data suggest that Crohn's disease (CD) results from dysregulation of the mucosal immune system in genetically predisposed individuals, leading to strong and ongoing activation of the immunological response to intestinal microflora [1].

What triggers the onset of CD is still an open question, despite the progress that has been made in defining the genetic and environmental risk factors and understanding the pathways linked to the immune response regarding the inflammation aspect of the pathology. Several pathways are proposed to drive the disease [2].

The overall inflammatory response in CD could be an additional risk factor responsible for the development of the disease. In this regard, specific molecular events that regulate the production of cytokines, such as the loss of function mutations in the genes encoding interleukin (IL)-10 and its receptor (IL-10R), can cause early onset of CD. In addition, the regressive inheritance of rare and low-frequency deleterious NOD2 variants contributes to 7–10% of CD cases [3].

The inflammatory response in CD is due to the balance between key pro- and anti-inflammatory cytokines: tumor necrosis factor alpha (TNFα), IFN-γ, interleukin (IL)-1, IL-18, IL-33, IL-36, and IL-38, which have pro-inflammatory effects, and IL-10, IL-4, IL-6, IL-11, IL-13, and transforming growth factor beta (TGF-β), which have anti-inflammatory effects [3].

The cardinal symptoms of CD are severe abdominal pain, diarrhea, bleeding, bowel obstruction, and a variety of systemic symptoms affecting the mouth, eyes, joints, and skin. For decades, aminosalicylates, immunosuppressive agents, and corticosteroids have been the standard of care for active CD to control inflammation and induce clinical remission. The biological drugs that target cytokines, such as anti-TNFα, JAK inhibitors, monoclonal α4β7 integrin antibody, and anti-IL-12/IL-23, are part of the armamentarium to obtain clinical and endoscopic remission.

Regarding therapy for CD, the route of administration, how to choose the first and second biologics, the potential of combination therapy with biologics, and the safety of biologics have been recently reported in several articles [4–6]. However, the use of anti-TNFα therapy has not yielded the expected declines in hospitalization and intestinal resection in IBD [7].

In the last decades, several pathogens (Table 1) have been found to have a role in the pathogenesis of CD [8,9], but only *E. coli* [10–13] and *Mycobacterium avium paratubercolosis* (MAP) [14,15] have aroused interest due to their strong association with CD pathogenesis. In 1998, a new pathovar strain of *E. coli*, defined as adherent invasive *E. coli* (AIEC), was isolated from the ileal mucosa of CD patients, as that was assumed to be a potential etiological source of the disease [16]. AIEC was found to adhere to gut epithelial cells, invade mucosa, penetrate and replicate into macrophages, and release inflammatory cytokines [13,17–19].

Table 1. Pathogens potentially involved in CD.

	Bacteria	References
✓	*Yersinia enterocolitica*	[2]
✓	*Helicobacter* species	[2]
✓	*Campylobacter* species	[2]
✓	*Listeria monocytogenes*	[2]
✓	*E. coli* species	[8–13]
✓	*Mycobacterium avium paratubercolosis*	[14,15]

It has been demonstrated that invasive *E. coli* strains isolated from CD patients are able to survive and replicate in large vacuoles within macrophages without inducing cell death. To survive and replicate in the harsh environment inside this compartment, AIEC strains utilize several adaptation mechanisms that permit them to resist phagocytosis and persist within macrophages, releasing large amounts of TNF-α [20].

Several independent studies, using different methods, reported an increased presence (from 25% to 55%) of mucosa-associated AIEC in CD patients [21–23]. AIEC was also recovered from 65% of chronic lesions and nearly 100% of biopsies from early lesions of CD patients [16]. In two recent reviews, AIEC was found in 23% and 29% of colonic mucosa biopsies from 69 and 304 CD patients, respectively [2,24]. All of these studies support the growing evidence that AIEC may be strongly involved in CD pathogenesis. Until now, few studies have been performed related to antibiotic treatment for active CD patients targeting AIEC. Unfortunately, the overall results are still scarce and unimpressive [25,26].

In addition to the presence of AIEC, several studies [27–29] reported the presence of MAP in intestinal biopsies of active CD patients, and for many years, it was also supposed that there may be an association between MAP and CD. Mycobacteria, like AIEC, survive and persist within host macrophages, and effective anti-mycobacterial agents require intracellular penetration.

Recently, Khan et al. [2], using the RT-PCR method, found a significantly increased prevalence of MAP (23.2%) in biopsy samples from CD patients compared with non-IBD controls. Mycobacterial tuberculosis and MAP show different antibiotic sensitivities [30]. Several anti-MAP trials have been performed, some using a single drug and others using up to four drugs [31]. Although some trials and several case reports described mucosal healing and eradication of MAP [32], randomized trials with anti-MAP antibiotic treatment did not show any prolonged benefit for CD patients [33–36].

Townsend et al. showed that the outcome of short-term antibiotic treatment, which is useful for induction and remission of active CD, was uncertain [37]. Long-term antibiotic treatment trials have been also performed, but several questions were raised about the factors that could limit the effectiveness of antibiotic treatment: trial design, duration of treatment, dose, and combination of antibiotics. Until now, the choice of antibiotic treatment has always been arbitrary, and the primary endpoint was clinical and endoscopic remission.

In this paper, we provide an overview and update of the data from trials on antibiotic treatment of active CD, taking into account the role of pathogens in the progression of the disease and the mechanism of action of different antibiotics on harmful pathogens. This review takes a brief look at the past, present, and future of antibiotic-based therapies for patients with active CD.

Since we cannot exclude that the etiopathogenesis of CD may involve AIEC in some cases and MAP in others, we suggest that the choice of antibiotic treatment for active CD needs to consider the target pathogens. In fact, if the cause of the pathology is the presence of a specific bacterial species, eradication of that species would necessarily be beneficial for the regression of inflammation.

In the end, we tried to present new lines of study for the use of antibiotics with personalized therapy for CD patients, taking into account the presence or absence of a specific bacterial species.

2. Literature Search Strategy

A literature search was conducted using the National Institute of Health (NIH) website (http://www.clinicaltrials.gov, accessed on 8 December 2023) focused on antibiotic treatment targeting MAP and AIEC as an intervention in human trials with CD patients. There were no restrictions regarding language, research location, and research race. We carried out the bibliographic search from 2002 to 2023.

The NIH database was chosen because it registers clinical trials around the world and the information is updated daily, and all of them are reviewed and approved by ethics committees or appropriate agencies and obey the appropriate national/state health agency regulations. We used an advanced search without any language restriction. The term "antibiotic Crohn" was entered into the search box. Studies that had no relation to antibiotic treatment were excluded.

3. Antibiotic Treatment Targeting MAP in Active CD Patients

Several meta-analyses have been published concerning long-term antibiotic treatment targeting MAP in patients with active CD (Table 2).

Table 2. Long-term antibiotic treatment targeting MAP in patients with active CD.

Author	Number of Trials	Number of Patients	Antibiotics	Duration	Placebo or Other Comparators	Primary Outcome	OR
Borgoankar [33]	6	317	Anti-MAP + corticosteroids (2 trials)	6–24 months	-	CDAI < 150	1.10 (0.69–1.74) (all trials)
		865	Anti-MAP + standard therapy (4 trials)				3.37 (1.38–8.24) (2 trials)
Feller [34]	16	58	Rifaximin (1 trial)	3 months	Placebo	CDAI < 150	2.07 (0.71–6.06)
		206	Nitroimidazole (3 trials)	3–24 months	Placebo	CDAI < 150	3.54 (1.94–6.47)
		322	Clofazimine (4 trials)	3–24 months	Placebo	CDAI > 70 from baseline	2.86 (1.67–4.88)
		287	Clarithromycin alone or in combination (4 trials)	3–24 months	Placebo	CDAI < 150	0.58 (0.29–1.18)
		107	Anti-tuberculosis drugs (3 trials)	3–24 months	Placebo	CDAI < 150	11.3 (2.60–48.8)
		47	Ciprofloxacin (1 trial)	6 months	Placebo	CDAI < 150	0.85 (0.73–0.99)
Khan [35]	10	1160	Macrolides, fluorochinolones, 5-nitromidazole, Rifaximin alone or in combination	1–4 months	Placebo	CDAI < 150	0.85
Selby [38]	1	213	Rifabutin, clarithromycin, and clofazimine (AMAT)	16–104 months	Placebo + 16 weeks tapering course Prednisolone	At least 1 relapse between 16 and 52 weeks	2.04 (0.84–4.93)
Graham [39]	1	331	RHB104: rifabutin, clarithromycin, or Clofazimine + anti-TNF or azatioprine or 6-mercaptopurine + 5 ASA corcorticosteroids (tapering after 8 weeks)	12 months	Placebo	CDAI < 150	at 26 weeks
Agrawal [40]	1	16	Rifabutin, clarithromycin, clofazimine + metronidazole or ciprofloxacin	5 months	-	wPCDAI: 47.5	-

OR, odds ratio; CDAI, Crohn's Disease Activity Index; and wPCDAI, Weighted Pediatric Crohn's Disease Activity Index.

Borgaonkar et al. [33] identified six randomized controlled trials (RCTs) using anti-MAP therapy for 6 to 24 months. Two trials that used corticosteroids in combination with antimicrobial therapy yielded a pooled odds ratio (OR) of 3.37 for maintenance of remission in treatment versus control, which was statistically significant (95% CI: 1.38–8.24; $p = 0.013$). The subgroup analysis of the other four trials, which did not use corticosteroids to induce remission, yielded a pooled odds ratio of 0.69 (95% CI: 0.39–1.21) for maintenance of remission in treatment versus control, which was not statistically significant ($p = 0.25$). The pooled OR for maintenance of remission in treatment versus control for all six studies was 1.10 (95% CI: 0.69–1.74) in favor of treatment, which was not statistically significant ($p = 0.78$). These results suggest that antimicrobial therapy is effective in maintaining remission in patients with CD after a course of corticosteroids combined with anti-MAP therapy.

Feller et al. [34], in a systematic review and meta-analysis of placebo-controlled trials, examined 13 treatment regimens in 865 patients. The average duration of treatment was 6 months. The outcomes were remission in patients with active disease and relapse in patients with inactive disease. The trials using nitroimidazoles showed benefits, with an OR of 3.54, and the OR for the four trials using clofazimine was 2.86. On the contrary, no benefit was found for classic drugs against tuberculosis (OR = 0.58). The results for clarithromycin were mixed ($p = 0.005$), and in three trials with rifaximin the OR was 2.07. The conclusion of this study was that long-term treatment with nitroimidazoles, clofazimine, or ciprofloxacin appeared to be effective in patients with active CD, while little evidence of benefits was found for clarithromycin and the classical tuberculosis drugs.

Khan et al. [35], in a systematic review including 10 RCTs and 1160 patients, evaluated the effect of antibiotics on remission and relapse of adult patients with active CD. Different kinds of antibiotics were tested, including macrolides, fluoroquinolones, 5-nitroimidazole, and rifaximin, either alone or in combination, for 4 to 16 weeks. There was a statistically significant effect of antibiotics on inducing remission in patients with active CD compared with placebo (OR = 0.85; 95% CI: 0.73–0.99).

Selby et al. [38], in a double-blind, placebo-controlled trial, studied 213 patients with active CD randomized to a 2-year course of daily clarithromycin, rifabutin, and clofazimine or placebo in addition to a 16-week course of prednisolone. The primary endpoint was at least one relapse by 12, 24, or 36 months. Of 122 patients who entered the maintenance phase, 39% who took antibiotics experienced at least one relapse between weeks 16 and 52, compared with 56% who took a placebo (OR = 2.04; p = 0.054). The differences between antibiotics and placebo were not statistically significant. The authors concluded that the study did not support a significant pathogenic role for MAP in most CD patients.

The Graham multicenter MAP US study [39] was the first global randomized trial to assess the efficacy of anti-MAP therapy (RHB-104) for 12 months in active CD patients. The anti-MAP therapy, in addition to standard therapy, demonstrated a clinically meaningful and statistically significant treatment effect in the protocol, in which the primary endpoint was defined as remission (CDAI < 150) at week 26, and the secondary endpoint was early remission at week 16 and durable remission through week 52. The remission rate with or without anti-TNF therapy at 26 weeks was significantly higher than placebo (37% vs. 23%, p = 0.07). At week 16, the remission rate was 42% vs. 29% (p = 0.015).

Agrawal et al. [40], studying a small cohort of pediatric CD patients, concluded that anti-MAP therapy may be more effective than the currently utilized therapies for inducing clinical and endoscopic remission. Although only 47% of patients achieved clinical remission by their first clinical follow-up, 93% of patients achieved remission by the subsequent follow-up appointments after an average of 5 months of treatment (p < 0.001).

Lastly, several case series have also been published concerning long-term antibiotic treatment targeting MAP [41,42]. In the Agrawal case series, CD patients experienced profound remission and required no further treatment for 3–23 years [41]. However, the trials and case series produced conflicting results, and no definitive conclusions could be drawn about the favorable effect of anti-MAP therapy on putative MAP infections in CD patients. Moreover, prophylactic antitubercular therapy was found to accelerate disease progression in patients with CD receiving anti-TNF-α therapy [43].

4. Antibiotic Treatment Targeting AIEC in Patients with Active CD

Most infections due to intracellular bacteria respond poorly to antibiotic treatment [44]. The lack of antibacterial activity is due to inactivation by the low pH of the phagolysosomes in which antimicrobial bacteria live [45]. Like *Coxiella burnetii*, *Tropheryma whipplei*, and several other bacteria, AIEC also replicates into macrophage phagolysosomes.

Wiseman et al. [46] first described the effect of pH on the inhibitory activity of chloroquine against *E. coli*. Recently, hydroxychloroquine (HCQ) was found to enhance antibiotic efficacy and macrophage killing of AIEC due to its alkalizing effect on the pH of phagolysosomes [47]. In a study by Flanagan [48], HCQ showed synergistic effects with doxycycline and ciprofloxacin, which are effective antibiotics against intracellular AIEC. Moreover, both HCQ and vitamin D caused dose-dependent inhibition of intramacrophagic AIEC replication 3 h after infection [48].

Rodhes et al. [49], in a randomized trial investigating the treatment of patients with active CD, evaluated prolonged antibiotic treatment with ciprofloxacin, doxycycline, and HCQ for 4 weeks followed by 20 weeks of doxycycline and HCQ, and compared antibiotics with budesonide treatment. The results, including crossover results, showed remission in 9 out of 24 patients treated with HCQ/antibiotics versus only 1 out of 32 patients treated with budesonide. Overall, the results on the efficacy of antibiotic treatment for AIEC-positive CD patients are still scarce and unimpressive. Further clinical trials will be necessary to assess the efficacy of combinations of antibiotics targeting AIEC.

5. Short-Term Antibiotic Treatment

Several RCTs utilizing short-term antibiotic treatment for induction and remission of CD produced conflicting results. Steinart et al. [50], analyzing RCTs including 134 patients treated with metronidazole and ciprofloxacin in combination with budesonide, found no differences in remission rates compared with placebo (OR = 1.02; CI: 0.62–1.66) (Table 3). Rahimi et al. [51], in a meta-analysis of broad-spectrum antibiotics, found that patients who received antibacterial therapy for 2 to 24 weeks were 2.257 times more likely to have clinical improvement than those who received placebo (Table 3). Six randomized placebo-controlled trials were included in the meta-analysis. Pulling the results from these trials yielded an OR of 2.157 (CI: 1.678–3.036) for antimicrobial therapy compared with placebo. The conclusion from this study was that broad-spectrum antibiotics improved clinical outcomes in patients with CD.

Table 3. Short-term antibiotic treatment for patients with active CD.

Author	Number of Trials	Number of Patients	Antibiotics	Duration	Placebo or Other Comparators	Primary Outcome	OR
Steinhart [50]	1	134	Metronidazole, ciprofloxacin, budesonide	8 weeks	Placebo	CDAI < 150	-
Rahimi [51]	6	804	Metronidazole, ciprofloxacin, Cotrimoxazole alone (2 trials) or in combination (4 trials)	2–24 weeks	Placebo	CDAI < 150	2.257
Prantera [52]	1	402	Rifaximin	12 weeks	Placebo	CDAI < 150	-
Wang [53]	-	83	Ciprofloxacin, metronuidazole alone or in combination, rifaximin, clarithromycin	2–16 weeks	Placebo	CDAI < 150	1.35
Su [54]	15	1407	Ciprofloxacin, fluoroquinolones, clarithromycin, metronidazole, rifaximin	at least 4 weeks	Placebo	CDAI < 15	1.35
Townsend [37]	13	1303	Rifaximin, clarithomycin, metronidazole, cotrimoxazole, Anti-MAP alone or in combination with budesonide	6–14 weeks	Placebo alone or in combination	CDAI < 150	0.77 to 0.33

OR, odds ratio; CDAI, Crohn's Disease Activity Index.

Prantera et al. [52] studied 402 CD patients after 12 weeks of rifaximin treatment in a clinical trial. After the treatment, 62% of the patients were in clinical remission ($p < 0.005$) (Table 3). Wang et al. [53], in a meta-analysis of broad-spectrum antibiotic therapy, noted clinical improvement in 56% of patients in the antibiotic group and 37.9% in the placebo group after 2–16 weeks of treatment (OR = 1.35 for clinical improvement) (Table 3). Su et al. [54], in a systematic review and meta-analysis, examined 1407 CD patients who received antibiotics for at least 4 weeks, including ciprofloxacin, clarithromycin, metronidazole, and rifaximin. Pooled analysis revealed that, compared with the placebo group, CD patients benefited to a certain extent (RR = 1.32; $p < 0.00001$). However, subgroup analysis showed that there was no significant difference between ciprofloxacin and control (Table 3). Townsend et al. [37] analyzed 13 eligible RCTs comparing antibiotics with a placebo or an active comparator in adult CD patients. Ciprofloxacin, rifaximin, metronidazole, clarithromycin, and cotrimoxazole, alone or in combination, provided only a modest benefit for the induction and maintenance of remission (OD ratio = 0.86 at 6–10 weeks and 0.77 at 10–14 weeks) (Table 3).

Due to the relatively low number of high-quality studies on antibiotics and the high variability in the tested antibiotics, treatment course, and outcome measures, drawing firm conclusions remains difficult.

6. Other Therapeutic Strategies Targeting AIEC

Since antimicrobial resistance was observed to affect antibiotics considered to be effective against intracellular AIEC, other possible strategies targeting AIEC have also been proposed:

- Anti-adhesive molecules

Monovalent mannosides are promising candidates for use in an alternative and complementary approach for CD patients colonized by AIEC [55]. Type-1 pili are utilized by Gram-negative bacteria to adhere to the host tissue and thus are a key virulence factor in CD. The type-1 pilus was found to mediate the recognition and attachment of AIEC strain to the host [56]. A mannoside recognizing Fim H adhesion, blocking the adhesion of bacteria to cells, was found in the type-1 pilus. A large panel of mannoside-derived Fim H antagonists has been tested to assess the ability of the antagonists to inhibit *E. coli* adhesion to host cells [57].

- Fecal microbiota transplantation

Fecal microbiota transplantation (FMT) is an emerging approach for IBD treatment to restore essential components of the intestinal flora. Modifying the microbial environment by FMT offers an alternative approach that could indirectly influence the host's immune system in a safe way. One of the newest and least explored methods of modifying the GI microbiota in IBD involves FMT. In the last decade, FMT has undergone a promising transformation, from being considered an alternative form of treatment lacking sufficient medical evidence to be held in reserve, to being accepted as a primary effective therapeutic option.

The FMT procedure involves transferring processed feces from a donor into the gastrointestinal tract of a patient. A recent systematic review and meta-analysis investigated 596 pediatric and adult IBD patients who were enrolled to receive FMT therapy [58]. The pooled estimated clinical remission for CD patients was 30% (CI: 11–52%).

Recently, the efficacy of FMT has been demonstrated in CD patients in independent studies [59–62]. In a systematic review and meta-analysis, Cheng et al. [63] evaluated the efficacy and safety of FMT treatment in CD patients. Twelve trials were analyzed: after FMT treatment, 0.62% of patients (CI: 0.48–0.51) achieved clinical remission and 0.79% (CI: 0.71–0.89) demonstrated a clinical response. Other adverse events were minor and resolved on their own.

- Probiotics, prebiotics, and postbiotics

The administration of probiotics with presumed anti-inflammatory activity has been tested in CD patients [64], and the efficacy and safety of probiotics for the induction and remission of CD have been reported. As reported in the Cochrane Database of Systematic Reviews [65], after 6 months of treatment there were no significant differences between probiotic treatment and placebo for the induction of remission in CD (OR = 1.06; CI: 0.65–1.71).

Colicin, a species-specific antibiotic, was also investigated. Colicin enters AIEC-containing vacuoles within macrophages and can be delivered either as a purified protein or through colic-producing bacteria. The use of *E. coli* Nissle 1917 as a colicin-producing prebiotic allowed the bacteria to secrete the selected colicin, which is toxic to the AIEC strain [66]. Colicin could potentially be useful to target specific pathogens such as AIEC, where maintaining a healthy microbiome is desirable.

- Phage therapy

Phage therapy is a biological treatment against bacterial infection; however, it targets only a limited number of bacterial strains. An interesting study showed that LF82-P2, LF82-P6, and LF82-P8 phages were effective against AIEC in a mouse model [67]. Galtier et al. [68] found that a single day of oral treatment with bacteriophages significantly decreased intestinal colonization by AIEC strain LF82. Phage therapy has been explored as a promising tool for the eradication of AIEC in CD [69]. Moreover, phage therapy against AIEC in CD patients was found to be safe and effective [70].

- Stem cells

Nowadays, stem cell therapy is widely used to treat CD. Although mesenchymal- and adipose-derived stem cells have proven to be safe for treating CD, there is still a lack of evidence on the efficacy of stem cell therapy for active CD. Moreover, there are still debates on the optimal protocol to use for such therapy in these patients. [71]. Recently, the mechanism of healing of CD patients after mesenchymal stem cell therapy has been reported.

7. Discussion

Based on the effectiveness of antibiotics as well as their favorable adverse effect profile and lower cost compared with biologic drugs or immunomodulators, they provide a more attractive therapeutic option for the treatment of moderate or severe active CD. Generally, traditional antibiotics have shown poor efficacy in active CD, so they are mostly indicated for treating septic complications in the postoperative setting. The rationale for using antibiotics as the primary treatment for CD is based on the increased evidence implicating gut bacteria in the pathogenesis of the disease. However, since the target organism and site of action (intracellular or extracellular) are unknown, the choice of antibiotics can only be arbitrary, and the use of a single antibiotic for short-term treatment can result in antibiotic resistance [44].

Overall, according to the *Antimicrobial consumption in the EU/EEA (ESAC-Net) Annual Epidemiological Report for 2021* [72], in the European Union, *E. coli* was the most common bacterial species (39.4%), with antimicrobial resistance in all reported cases. Antimicrobial agents such as penicillins, cephalosporins, and aminoglycosides, which penetrate poorly into macrophages, are generally ineffective against diseases induced by pathogens that are present within macrophages (Figure 1). On the contrary, azithromycin, ciprofloxacin, clarithromycin, rifampin, sulfamethoxazole, tetracycline, and trimethoprim have been shown to be effective against pathogens such as *E. coli* and MAP internalized by macrophages (Figure 1).

For these reasons, combination therapy using antibiotics that penetrate macrophages may provide a more effective treatment when targeting AIEC [73]. It has been reported that the acid condition of phagolysosomes, in which *E. coli* is located, inhibits antibiotic activity. HCQ, an alkalinizing agent, demonstrated synergistic effects with doxycycline and ciprofloxacin, enhancing the antibiotic efficacy against intramacrophagic AIEC [47,48]. Rodhes et al. [49] found no significant differences in remission or response rates between the antibiotic/HCQ combination and a standard 12-week course of budesonide at 10, 24, or 52 weeks when assessed by intention-to-treat analysis. In that study, to eradicate AIEC in CD patients, ciprofloxacin was used only for 4 weeks and doxycycline was used alone for 20 weeks, which is too short a time to obtain a favorable response. It is our opinion that the unfavorable results of Rhodes's trial were due to antibiotic resistance.

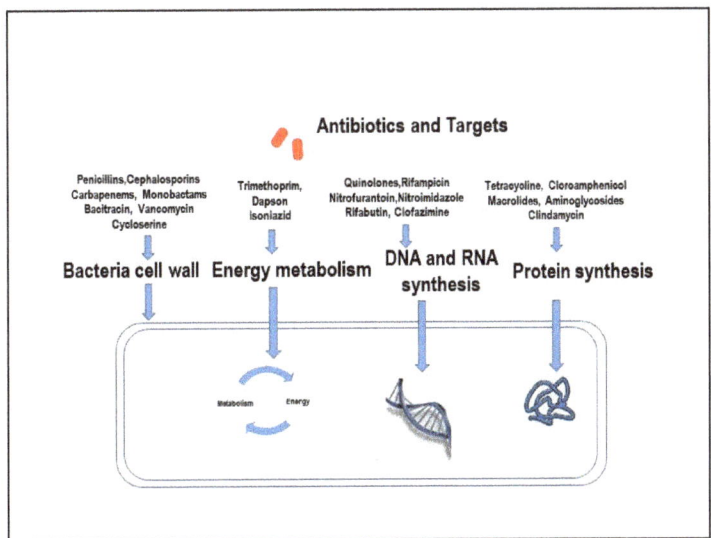

Figure 1. Mechanisms by which antibiotics act on harmful pathogens.

Dogan et al. [74] showed that AIEC resistance to one or more antimicrobial agents was present in 75% of CD patients colonized with AIEC and 60% of patients with normal ileum colonized with AIEC ($p < 0.05$). None of the strains were simultaneously resistant to ciprofloxacin, tetracycline, and trimethoprim. AIEC resistance to ciprofloxacin, tetracycline, clarithromycin, rifampicin, and trimethoprim–sulfamethoxazole was found in 25%, 50%, 37.5%, 37.5%, and 50% of CD patients colonized with AIEC, respectively [73].

According to a review by Ledder and Turner, the use of ciprofloxacin with or without metronidazole in perianal CD could be valuable as an adjunct to biologics; once again, metronidazole offered benefit in preventing postoperative recurrence in CD patients [75].

It has also been supposed for years that there may be an association between MAP and CD. Several RCTs showed favorable but conflicting results regarding the clinical remission of CD patients after prolonged therapy with multiple anti-MAP drugs [39–41]. Unfortunately, in a few trials, MAP detection was performed before treatment, often using inconsistent methods such as culture techniques, which have many limitations, including poor sensitivity. Moreover, in all trials, the primary endpoint of antibiotic treatment was always clinical and endoscopic remission or relapse, evaluated by CDAI and SES-CD.

8. Conclusions

In light of the data in the literature, we cannot exclude the notion that the etiopathogenesis of some CD patients may be due to AIEC in some cases and MAP in others, and that the choice of antibiotic treatment for patients with active CD needs to consider the target pathogens. In patients with active CD colonized by AIEC or MAP, a combination of antibiotics that penetrate macrophages should be administered for at least 6 months to avoid antimicrobial resistance. The primary treatment endpoint should be the eradication of pathogens. The secondary endpoint could be clinical and endoscopic remission according to CDAI and SES-CD.

9. Future Directions

For all patients with a new diagnosis of CD based on clinical and endoscopic findings, we recommend the detection of AIEC and MAP in ileal/colonic mucosal biopsies using RT-PCR. In patients with active CD and associated AIEC, antibiotic therapy could be administered as a combination of multiple macrophage-penetrating antibiotics. To avoid antibiotic resistance, HCQ could also be used in combination with ciprofloxacin, tetracycline, and trimethoprim for at least 6 months (Figure 2).

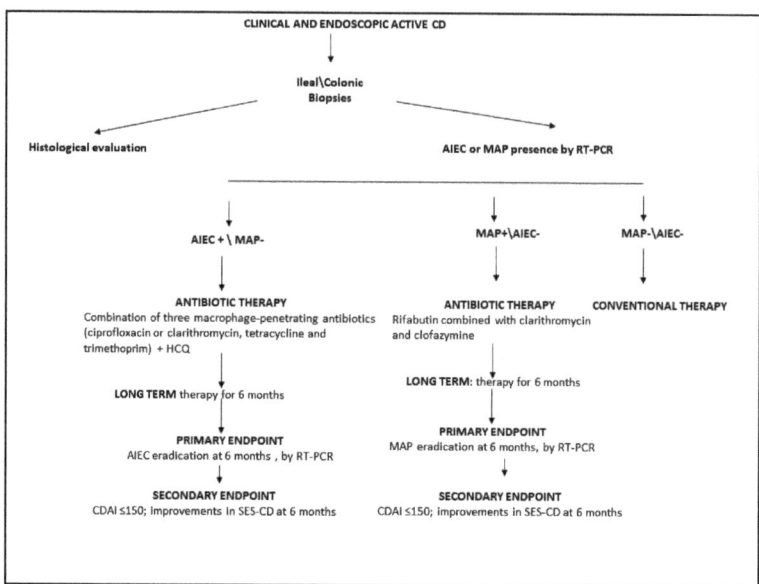

Figure 2. Schematic workflow for antibiotic treatment of patients with active CD. HCQ, hydroxychloroquine; AIEC, adherent invasive *E. coli*; MAP, *Mycobacterium avium paratuberculosis*; CDAI, Crohn's Disease Activity Index; SES-CD, Simple Endoscopic Score for Crohn's Disease; RT-PCR, real-time polymerase chain reaction.

For patients with active CD and associated MAP, we suggest long-term (up to 6 months) anti-MAP treatment with rifabutin, clarithromycin, and clofazimine (Figure 2). For all CD patients colonized with AIEC or MAP treated with antimicrobial therapy, the primary treatment endpoint should be the eradication of AIEC or MAP, as assessed by RT-PCR (Figure 2). The secondary endpoint should be clinical and endoscopic remission, as evaluated by CDAI and SES CD.

Finally, conventional therapy could be suggested only for CD patients without associated AIEC or MAP (Figure 2).

Author Contributions: Conceptualization and draft, G.I.; writing—review and editing, V.R.A.; review, editing, and supervision, C.S., G.M., A.D.L., S.I., A.L. and R.M. All authors have read and agreed to the published version of the manuscript.

Funding: This research received no external funding.

Conflicts of Interest: The authors declare no conflicts of interest.

References

1. Roda, G.; Chien Ng, S.; Kotze, P.G.; Argollo, M.; Panaccione, R.; Spinelli, A.; Kaser, A.; Peyrin-Biroulet, L.; Danese, S. Crohn's disease. *Nat. Rev. Dis. Primers* **2020**, *6*, 26, Erratum in *Nat. Rev. Dis. Primers* **2020**, *6*, 22. [CrossRef]
2. Khan, I.A.; Nayak, B.; Markandey, M.; Bajaj, A.; Verma, M.; Kumar, S.; Singh, M.K.; Kedia, S.; Ahuja, V. Differential prevalence of pathobionts and host gene polymorphisms in chronic inflammatory intestinal diseases: Crohn's disease and intestinal tuberculosis. *PLoS ONE* **2021**, *16*, e0256098. [CrossRef] [PubMed]
3. Vebr, M.; Pomahačová, R.; Sýkora, J.; Schwarz, J. A Narrative Review of Cytokine Networks: Pathophysiological and Therapeutic Implications for Inflammatory Bowel Disease Patho-genesis. *Biomedicines* **2023**, *11*, 3229. [CrossRef] [PubMed]

4. Queiroz, N.S.F.; Barros, L.L.; Azevedo, M.F.C.; Oba, J.; Sobrado, C.W.; Carlos, A.S.; Milani, L.R.; Sipahi, A.M.; Damião, A.O.M.C. Management of inflammatory bowel disease patients in the COVID-19 pandemic era: A Brazilian tertiary referral center guidance. *Clinics* 2020, *75*, e1909. [CrossRef]
5. Liefferinckx, C.; Cremer, A.; Franchimont, D. Switching biologics used in inflammatory bowel diseases: How to deal with in practice? *Curr. Opin. Pharmacol.* 2020, *55*, 82–89. [CrossRef] [PubMed]
6. Colombel, J.F.; Panaccione, R.; Bossuyt, P.; Lukas, M.; Baert, F.; Vaňásek, T.; Danalioglu, A.; Novacek, G.; Armuzzi, A.; Hébuterne, X.; et al. Effect of tight control management on Crohn's disease (CALM): A multicentre, randomised, controlled phase 3 trial. *Lancet* 2017, *390*, 2779–2789, Erratum in *Lancet* 2018, *390*, 2768. [CrossRef] [PubMed]
7. Murthy, S.K.; Begum, J.; Benchimol, E.I.; Bernstein, C.N.; Kaplan, G.G.; McCurdy, J.D.; Singh, H.; Targownik, L.; Taljaard, M. Introduction of anti-TNF therapy has not yielded expected declines in hospitalisation and intestinal resection rates in inflammatory bowel diseases: A population-based interrupted time series study. *Gut* 2020, *69*, 274–282. [CrossRef]
8. Ahmed, M.; Metwaly, A.; Haller, D. Modeling microbe-host interaction in the pathogenesis of Crohn's disease. *Int. J. Med. Microbiol.* 2021, *311*, 151489. [CrossRef]
9. Iaquinto, G.; Rotondi Aufiero, V.; Mazzarella, G.; Lucariello, A.; Panico, L.; Melina, R.; Iaquinto, S.; De Luca, A.; Sellitto, C. Pathogens in Crohn's disease: The role of Adherent Invasive *Escherichia coli*. *Crit. Rev. Eukaryot. Gene Expr.* 2024, *34*, 83–99. [CrossRef]
10. Mirsepasi-Lauridsen, H.C.; Vallance, B.A.; Krogfelt, K.A.; Petersen, A.M. *Escherichia coli* Pathobionts Associated with Inflammatory Bowel Disease. *Clin. Microbiol. Rev.* 2019, *32*, e00060-18. [CrossRef]
11. Palmela, C.; Chevarin, C.; Xu, Z.; Torres, J.; Sevrin, G.; Hirten, R.; Barnich, N.; Ng, S.C.; Colombel, J.F. Adherent-invasive *Escherichia coli* in inflammatory bowel disease. *Gut* 2018, *67*, 574–587. [CrossRef]
12. Shaler, C.R.; Elhenawy, W.; Coombes, B.K. The Unique Lifestyle of Crohn's Disease-Associated Adherent-Invasive *Escherichia coli*. *J. Mol. Biol.* 2019, *431*, 2970–2981. [CrossRef]
13. Zheng, L.; Duan, S.L.; Dai, Y.C.; Wu, S.C. Role of adherent invasive *Escherichia coli* in pathogenesis of inflammatory bowel disease. *World J. Clin. Cases* 2022, *10*, 11671–11689. [CrossRef]
14. Agrawal, G.; Aitken, J.; Hamblin, H.; Collins, M.; Borody, T.J. Putting Crohn's on the MAP: Five Common Questions on the Contribution of Mycobacterium avium subspecies paratuberculosis to the Pathophysiology of Crohn's Disease. *Dig. Dis. Sci.* 2021, *66*, 348–358. [CrossRef]
15. Aitken, J.M.; Phan, K.; Bodman, S.E.; Sharma, S.; Watt, A.; George, P.M.; Agrawal, G.; Tie, A.B.M. A Mycobacterium species for Crohn's disease? *Pathology* 2021, *53*, 818–823. [CrossRef]
16. Darfeuille-Michaud, A.; Neut, C.; Barnich, N.; Lederman, E.; Di Martino, P.; Desreumaux, P.; Gambiez, L.; Joly, B.; Cortot, A.; Colombel, J.F. Presence of adherent *Escherichia coli* strains in ileal mucosa of patients with Crohn's disease. *Gastroenterology* 1998, *115*, 1405–1413. [CrossRef] [PubMed]
17. Mazzarella, G.; Perna, A.; Marano, A.; Lucariello, A.; Rotondi Aufiero, V.; Sorrentino, A.; Melina, R.; Guerra, G.; Taccone, F.S.; Iaquinto, G.; et al. Pathogenic Role of Associated Adherent-Invasive *Escherichia coli* in Crohn's Disease. *J. Cell. Physiol.* 2017, *232*, 2860–2868. [CrossRef] [PubMed]
18. Lee, J.G.; Han, D.S.; Jo, S.V.; Lee, A.R.; Park, C.H.; Eun, C.S.; Lee, Y. Characteristics and pathogenic role of adherent-invasive *Escherichia coli* in inflammatory bowel disease: Potential impact on clinical outcomes. *PLoS ONE* 2019, *14*, e0216165. [CrossRef]
19. Mansour, S.; Asrar, T.; Elhenawy, W. The multifaceted virulence of adherent-invasive *Escherichia coli*. *Gut Microbes* 2023, *15*, 2172669. [CrossRef] [PubMed]
20. Glasser, A.L.; Boudeau, J.; Barnich, N.; Perruchot, M.H.; Colombel, J.F.; Darfeuille-Michaud, A. Adherent invasive *Escherichia coli* strains from patients with Crohn's disease survive and replicate within macrophages without inducing host cell death. *Infect. Immun.* 2001, *69*, 5529–5537. [CrossRef] [PubMed]
21. Campbell, J.; Borody, T.J.; Leis, S. The many faces of Crohn's disease: Latest concepts in etiology. *Open J. Int. Med.* 2012, *2*, 107. [CrossRef]
22. Darfeuille-Michaud, A.; Boudeau, J.; Bulois, P.; Neut, C.; Glasser, A.L.; Barnich, N.; Bringer, M.A.; Swidsinski, A.; Beaugerie, L.; Colombel, J.F. High prevalence of adherent-invasive *Escherichia coli* associated with ileal mucosa in Crohn's disease. *Gastroenterology* 2004, *127*, 412–421. [CrossRef]
23. Buisson, A.; Vazeille, E.; Fumery, M.; Pariente, B.; Nancey, S.; Seksik, P.; Peyrin-Biroulet, L.; Allez, M.; Ballet, N.; Filippi, J.; et al. Faster and less invasive tools to identify patients with ileal colonization by adherent-invasive *E. coli* in Crohn's disease. *United Eur. Gastroenterol. J.* 2021, *9*, 1007–1018. [CrossRef]
24. Nadalian, B.; Yadegar, A.; Houri, H.; Olfatifar, M.; Shahrokh, S.; Asadzadeh Aghdaei, H.; Suzuki, H.; Zali, M.R. Prevalence of the pathobiont adherent-invasive *Escherichia coli* and inflammatory bowel disease: A systematic review and meta-analysis. *J. Gastroenterol. Hepatol.* 2021, *36*, 852–863. [CrossRef]
25. Petersen, A.M. Gastrointestinal dysbiosis and *Escherichia coli* pathobionts in inflammatory bowel diseases. *APMIS* 2022, *130* (Suppl. S144), 1–38. [CrossRef]
26. Spaulding, C.N.; Klein, R.D.; Schreiber, H.L., 4th; Janetka, J.W.; Hultgren, S.J. Precision antimicrobial therapeutics: The path of least resistance? *NPJ Biofilms Microbiomes* 2018, *4*, 4. [CrossRef]

27. Olsen, I.; Tollefsen, S.; Aagaard, C.; Reitan, L.J.; Bannantine, J.P.; Andersen, P.; Sollid, L.M.; Lundin, K.E. Isolation of Mycobacterium avium subspecies paratuberculosis reactive CD4 T cells from intestinal biopsies of Crohn's disease patients. *PLoS ONE* **2009**, *5*, e5641. [CrossRef] [PubMed]
28. Naser, S.A.; Sagramsingh, S.R.; Naser, A.S.; Thanigachalam, S. Mycobacterium avium subspecies paratuberculosis causes Crohn's disease in some inflammatory bowel disease patients. *World J. Gastroenterol.* **2014**, *20*, 7403–7415. [CrossRef] [PubMed]
29. Autschbach, F.; Eisold, S.; Hinz, U.; Zinser, S.; Linnebacher, M.; Giese, T.; Löffler, T.; Büchler, M.W.; Schmidt, J. High prevalence of Mycobacterium avium subspecies paratuberculosis IS900 DNA in gut tissues from individuals with Crohn's disease. *Gut* **2005**, *54*, 944–949. [CrossRef] [PubMed]
30. Greenstein, R.J. Is Crohn's disease caused by a mycobacterium? Comparisons with le-prosy, tuberculosis, and Johne's disease. *Lancet Infect. Dis.* **2003**, *3*, 507–514. [CrossRef] [PubMed]
31. Mintz, M.J.; Lukin, D.J. Mycobacterium avium subspecies paratuberculosis (MAP) and Crohn's disease: The debate continues. *Transl. Gastroenterol. Hepatol.* **2023**, *8*, 28. [CrossRef]
32. Chamberlin, W.; Borody, T.J.; Campbell, J. Primary treatment of Crohn's disease: Combi-ned antibiotics taking center stage. *Expert. Rev. Clin. Immunol.* **2011**, *7*, 751–760. [CrossRef]
33. Borgaonkar, M.R.; MacIntosh, D.G.; Fardy, J.M. A meta-analysis of anti mycobacterial therapy for Crohn's disease. *Am. J. Gastroenterol.* **2000**, *95*, 725–729. [CrossRef] [PubMed]
34. Feller, M.; Huwiler, K.; Schoepfer, A.; Shang, A.; Furrer, H.; Egger, M. Long-term antibiotic treatment for Crohn's disease: Systematic review and me-ta-analysis of placebo-controlled trials. *Clin. Infect. Dis.* **2010**, *50*, 473–480. [CrossRef] [PubMed]
35. Khan, K.J.; Ullman, T.A.; Ford, A.C.; Abreu, M.T.; Abadir, A.; Marshall, J.K.; Talley, N.J.; Moayyedi, P. Antibiotic therapy in inflammatory bowel disease: A systematic review and meta-analysis. *Am. J. Gastroenterol.* **2011**, *106*, 661–673, Erratum in *Am. J. Gastroenterol.* **2011**, *106*, 1014. [CrossRef] [PubMed]
36. Savarino, E.; Bertani, L.; Ceccarelli, L.; Bodini, G.; Zingone, F.; Buda, A.; Facchin, S.; Lorenzon, G.; Marchi, S.; Marabotto, E.; et al. Antimicrobial treatment with the fixed-dose antibiotic combination RHB-104 for Mycobacterium avium subspecies paratuberculosis in Crohn's disease: Pharmacological and clinical implications. *Expert Opin. Biol. Ther.* **2019**, *19*, 79–88. [CrossRef] [PubMed]
37. Townsend, C.M.; Parker, C.E.; MacDonald, J.K.; Nguyen, T.M.; Jairath, V.; Feagan, B.G.; Khanna, R. Antibiotics for induction and maintenance of remission in Crohn's disease. *Cochrane Database Syst. Rev.* **2019**, *2*, CD012730. [CrossRef] [PubMed]
38. Selby, W.; Pavli, P.; Crotty, B.; Florin, T.; Radford-Smith, G.; Gibson, P.; Mitchell, B.; Connell, W.; Read, R.; Merrett, M.; et al. Antibiotics in Crohn's Disease Study Group. Two-year combination antibiotic therapy with clarithromycin, rifabutin, and clofazimine for Crohn's disease. *Gastroenterology* **2007**, *132*, 2313–2319. [CrossRef] [PubMed]
39. Graham, D.; Naser, S.; Offman, E.; Nastya, K.; Robert, H.; Thomas, W.; Grazyna, R.; Beata, S.; Tomasz, A.; Wos Anna, W.; et al. RHB-104, a Fixed-Dose, Oral Antibiotic Combination Against Mycobacterium Avium Paratuberculosis (MAP) Infection, Is Effective in Moderately to Severely Active Crohn's Disease. *Am. J. Gastroenterol. Oct.* **2019**, *114*, S376–S377. [CrossRef]
40. Agrawal, G.; Hamblin, H.; Clancy, A.; Borody, T. Anti-Mycobacterial Antibiotic Therapy Induces Remission in Active Paediatric Crohn's Disease. *Microorganisms* **2020**, *8*, 1112. [CrossRef]
41. Agrawal, G.; Clancy, A.; Huynh, R.; Borody, T. Profound remission in Crohn's disease requiring no further treatment for 3–23 years: A case series. *Gut Pathog.* **2020**, *12*, 16. [CrossRef]
42. Honap, S.; Johnston, E.L.; Agrawal, G.; Al-Hakim, B.; Hermon-Taylor, J.; Sanderson, J.D. Anti-Mycobacterium paratuberculosis (MAP) therapy for Crohn's disease: An overview and update. *Frontline Gastroenterol.* **2020**, *12*, 397–403. [CrossRef]
43. Liu, F.; Tang, J.; Ye, L.; Tan, J.; Qiu, Y.; Hu, F.; He, J.; Chen, B.; He, Y.; Zeng, Z.; et al. Prophylactic Antitubercular Therapy Is Associated With Accelerated Disease Progression in Patients With Crohn's Disease Receiving Anti-TNF Therapy: A Retrospective Multicenter Study. *Clin. Transl. Gastroenterol.* **2022**, *13*, e00493. [CrossRef]
44. Demarre, G.; Prudent, V.; Schenk, H.; Rousseau, E.; Bringer, M.A.; Barnich, N.; Tran Van Nhieu, G.; Rimsky, S.; De Monte, S.; Espéli, O. The Crohn's disease-associated *Escherichia coli* strain LF82 relies on SOS and stringent responses to survive, multiply and tolerate antibiotics within macrophages. *PLoS Pathog.* **2019**, *15*, e1008123. [CrossRef]
45. Munita, J.M.; Arias, C.A. Mechanisms of Antibiotic Resistance. *Microbiol. Spectr.* **2016**, *4*, 464–473. [CrossRef]
46. Wiseman, D. The effect of pH on the inhibitory activity of chloroquine against *Esche-richia coli*. *J. Pharm. Pharmacol.* **1972**, *24*, 162p.
47. Flanagan, P.K.; Campbell, B.J.; Rhodes, J.M. Hydroxychloroquine as a treatment for Crohn's disease: Enhancing antibiotic efficacy and macrophage killing of *E coli*. *Gut* **2012**, *61*, A60–A61. [CrossRef]
48. Flanagan, P.K.; Chiewchengchol, D.; Wright, H.L.; Edwards, S.W.; Alswied, A.; Satsangi, J.; Subramanian, S.; Rhodes, J.M.; Campbell, B.J. Killing of *Escherichia coli* by Crohn's Disease Monocyte-derived Macrophages Its Enhancement by Hydroxychloroquine Vitamin, D. *Inflamm. Bowel Dis.* **2015**, *21*, 1499–1510. [CrossRef] [PubMed]
49. Rhodes, J.M.; Subramanian, S.; Flanagan, P.K.; Horgan, G.W.; Martin, K.; Mansfield, J.; Parkes, M.; Hart, A.; Dallal, H.; Iqbal, T.; et al. Randomized Trial of Ciprofloxacin Doxycycline and Hydroxychloroquine Versus Budesonide in Active Crohn's Disease. *Dig. Dis. Sci.* **2021**, *66*, 2700–2711. [CrossRef] [PubMed]
50. Steinhart, A.H.; Feagan, B.G.; Wong, C.J.; Vandervoort, M.; Mikolainis, S.; Croitoru, K.; Seidman, E.; Leddin, D.J.; Bitton, A.; Drouin, E.; et al. Combined budesonide and antibiotic therapy for active Crohn's disease: A randomized controlled trial. *Gastroenterology* **2002**, *123*, 33–40. [CrossRef] [PubMed]

51. Rahimi, R.; Nikfar, S.; Rezaie, A.; Abdollahi, M. A meta-analysis of broad-spectrum anti-biotic therapy in patients with active Crohn's disease. *Clin. Ther.* **2006**, *28*, 1983–1988. [CrossRef]
52. Prantera, C.; Lochs, H.; Grimaldi, M.; Danese, S.; Scribano, M.L.; Gionchetti, P.; Retic Study Group (Rifaximin-Eir Treatment in Crohn's Disease). Rifaximin-extended intestinal release induces remission in patients with moderately active Crohn's disease. *Gastroenterology* **2012**, *142*, 473–481.e4. [CrossRef]
53. Wang, S.L.; Wang, Z.R.; Yang, C.Q. Meta-analysis of broad-spectrum antibiotic therapy in patients with active inflammatory bowel disease. *Exp. Ther. Med.* **2012**, *4*, 1051–1056. [CrossRef]
54. Su, J.W.; Ma, J.J.; Zhang, H.J. Use of antibiotics in patients with Crohn's disease: A syste-matic review and meta-analysis. *J. Dig. Dis.* **2015**, *16*, 58–66. [CrossRef]
55. Sivignon, A.; Bouckaert, J.; Bernard, J.; Gouin, S.G.; Barnich, N. The potential of FimH as a novel therapeutic target for the treatment of Crohn's disease. *Expert Opin. Ther. Targets* **2017**, *21*, 837–847. [CrossRef]
56. Barnich, N.; Carvalho, F.A.; Glasser, A.L.; Darcha, C.; Jantscheff, P.; Allez, M.; Peeters, H.; Bommelaer, G.; Desreumaux, P.; Colombel, J.F.; et al. CEACAM6 acts as a receptor for adherent-invasive *E. coli*, supporting ileal mucosa colonization in Crohn disease. *J. Clin. Investig.* **2007**, *117*, 1566–1574. [CrossRef] [PubMed]
57. Mydock-McGrane, L.K.; Hannan, T.J.; Janetka, J.W. Rational design strategies for FimH antagonists: New drugs on the horizon for urinary tract infection and Crohn's disease. *Expert Opin. Drug Discov.* **2017**, *12*, 711–731. [CrossRef] [PubMed]
58. Fang, H.; Fu, L.; Wang, J. Protocol for Fecal Microbiota Transplantation in Inflammatory Bowel Disease: A Systematic Review and Meta-Analysis. *BioMed Res. Int.* **2018**, *2018*, 8941340. [CrossRef] [PubMed]
59. Gordon, H.; Harbord, M. A patient with severe Crohn's colitis responds to Faecal Microbiota Transplantation. *J. Crohn's Colitis* **2014**, *8*, 256–257. [CrossRef]
60. Cui, B.; Feng, Q.; Wang, H.; Wang, M.; Peng, Z.; Li, P.; Huang, G.; Liu, Z.; Wu, P.; Fan, Z.; et al. Fecal microbiota transplantation through mid-gut for refractory Crohn's disease: Safety, feasibility, and efficacy trial results. *J. Gastroenterol. Hepatol.* **2015**, *30*, 51–58. [CrossRef] [PubMed]
61. Kao, D.; Hotte, N.; Gillevet, P.; Madsen, K. Fecal micro-biota transplantation inducing remission in Crohn's colitis and the associated changes in fecal microbial profile. *J. Clin. Gastroenterol.* **2014**, *48*, 625–628. [CrossRef] [PubMed]
62. Vermeire, S.; Joossens, M.; Verbeke, K.; Hildebrand, F.; Machiels, K.; Van den Broeck, K.; Van Assche, G.; Rutgeerts, P.; Raes, J. Pilot Study on the safety and efficacy of faecal microbiota transplantation in refractory Crohn's disease. *Gastroenterology* **2012**, *142*, S360. [CrossRef]
63. Cheng, F.; Huang, Z.; Wei, W.; Li, Z. Fecal microbiota transplantation for Crohn's disease: A systematic review and me-ta-analysis. *Tech. Coloproctology* **2021**, *25*, 495–504. [CrossRef] [PubMed]
64. Tsilingiri, K.; Rescigno, M. Postbiotics: What else? *Benef. Microbes* **2013**, *4*, 101–107. [CrossRef] [PubMed]
65. Limketkai, B.N.; Akobeng, A.K.; Gordon, M.; Adepoju, A.A. Probiotics for in-duction of remission in Crohn's disease. *Cochrane Database Syst. Rev.* **2020**, *7*, CD006634. [CrossRef] [PubMed]
66. Kotłowski, R. Use of *Escherichia coli* Nissle 1917 producing recombinant colicins for treatment of IBD patients. *Med. Hypotheses* **2016**, *93*, 8–10. [CrossRef] [PubMed]
67. Sivignon, A.; Chervy, M.; Chevarin, C.; Ragot, E.; Billard, E.; Denizot, J.; Barnich, N. An adherent-invasive *Escherichia coli*-colonized mouse model to evaluate microbiota-targeting strategies in Crohn's disease. *Dis. Model. Mech.* **2022**, *15*, dmm049707. [CrossRef]
68. Galtier, M.; De Sordi, L.; Sivignon, A.; de Vallée, A.; Maura, D.; Neut, C.; Rahmouni, O.; Wannerberger, K.; Darfeuille-Michaud, A.; Desreumaux, P.; et al. Bacteriophages Targeting Adherent Invasive *Escherichia coli* Strains as a Promising New Treatment for Crohn's Disease. *J. Crohn's Colitis* **2017**, *11*, 840–847. [CrossRef]
69. Gutiérrez, B.; Domingo-Calap, P. Phage Therapy in Gastrointestinal Diseas-es. *Microorganisms* **2020**, *8*, 1420. [CrossRef]
70. Boucher, D.; Barnich, N. Phage Therapy Against Adherent-invasive *E. coli*: Towards a Promising Treatment of Crohn's Disease Patients? *J. Crohn's Colitis* **2022**, *16*, 1509–1510. [CrossRef]
71. Mohammadi, T.C.; Jazi, K.; Bolouriyan, A.; Soleymanitabar, A. Stem cells in treatment of crohn's disease: Recent advances and future directions. *Transpl. Immunol.* **2023**, *80*, 101903. [CrossRef]
72. WHO Regional Office for Europe/European Centre for Disease Prevention and Control. *An-Timicrobial Resistance Surveillance in Europe 2022–2020 Data*; WHO Regional Office for Europe: Copenhagen, Denmark, 2022.
73. Subramanian, S.; Roberts, C.L.; Hart, C.A.; Martin, H.M.; Edwards, S.W.; Rhodes, J.M.; Campbell, B.J. Replication of Colonic Crohn's Disease Mucosal *Escherichia coli* Isolates within Macrophages and Their Susceptibility to Antibiotics. *Antimicrob. Agents Chemother.* **2008**, *52*, 427–434. [CrossRef] [PubMed]
74. Dogan, B.; Scherl, E.; Bosworth, B.; Yantiss, R.; Altier, C.; McDonough, P.L.; Jiang, Z.D.; Dupont, H.L.; Garneau, P.; Harel, J.; et al. Multidrug resistance is common in *Escherichia coli* associated with ileal Crohn's disease. *Inflamm. Bowel Dis.* **2013**, *19*, 141–150. [CrossRef] [PubMed]
75. Ledder, O.; Turner, D. Antibiotics in IBD: Still a Role in the Biological Era? *Inflamm. Bowel Dis.* **2018**, *24*, 1676–1688. [CrossRef] [PubMed]

Disclaimer/Publisher's Note: The statements, opinions and data contained in all publications are solely those of the individual author(s) and contributor(s) and not of MDPI and/or the editor(s). MDPI and/or the editor(s) disclaim responsibility for any injury to people or property resulting from any ideas, methods, instructions or products referred to in the content.

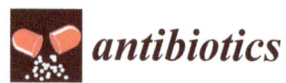

Article

Cefto Real-Life Study: Real-World Data on the Use of Ceftobiprole in a Multicenter Spanish Cohort

Carmen Hidalgo-Tenorio [1,*,†], Inés Pitto-Robles [1], Daniel Arnés García [1], F. Javier Membrillo de Novales [2], Laura Morata [3], Raul Mendez [4], Olga Bravo de Pablo [5], Vicente Abril López de Medrano [6], Miguel Salavert Lleti [7], Pilar Vizcarra [8], Jaime Lora-Tamayo [9], Ana Arnáiz García [10], Leonor Moreno Núñez [11], Mar Masiá [12], Maria Pilar Ruiz Seco [13] and Svetlana Sadyrbaeva-Dolgova [14]

1. Unit of Infectious Diseases, Hospital Universitario Virgen de las Nieves, Instituto de Investigación Biosanitario de Granada (IBS-Granada), 18012 Granada, Spain; ipittorobles@gmail.com (I.P.-R.); arnesgarciadaniel@gmail.com (D.A.G.)
2. CBRN and Infectious Diseases, Hospital General Defensa Gómez Ulla, 28047 Madrid, Spain; javimembrillo@gmail.com
3. Infectious Diseases Service, Hospital Clinic, 08036 Barcelona, Spain; lmorata@clinic.cat
4. Pneumology Deparment, Hospital Universitario La Fe, Valencia (CIBERES), 46026 Valencia, Spain; rmendezalcoy@gmail.com
5. Internal Medicine Service, Hospital La Moraleja, 28050 Madrid, Spain; olgabravodepablo@gmail.com
6. Infectious Diseases Service, Hospital General of Valencia, 46014 Valencia, Spain; vicente.abril.lopezdemedrano@gmail.com
7. Infectious Diseases Service, Hospital Universitario La Fe, Valencia (CIBERES), 46026 Valencia, Spain; salavert_mig@gva.es
8. Infectious Diseases Service, Hospital Ramón y Cajal, 28034 Madrid, Spain; pilar1vizcarra@gmail.com
9. Internal Medicine Service, Hospital Universitario 12 Octubre (CIBERINFEC), 28041 Madrid, Spain; sirsilverdelea@yahoo.com
10. Department of Infectious Diseases, Hospital Sierrallana, 39300 Torrelavega, Spain; anam.arnaiz@scsalud.es
11. Internal Medicine Service, Hospital Fundación de Alcorcón, 28922 Alcorcón, Spain; lmorenon@salud.madrid.org
12. Infectious Diseases Service, Hospital Universitario General of Elche, 03203 Elche, Spain; marmasiac@gmail.com
13. Internal Medicine Service, Hospital Infanta Sofía, 28702 Madrid, Spain; mprseco@salud.madrid.org
14. Pharmacy Service, Hospital Universitario Virgen de las Nieves, Instituto de Investigación Biosanitario de Granada (IBS-Granada), 18012 Granada, Spain; sadyrbaeva@gmail.com
* Correspondence: chidalgo72@gmail.com; Tel.: +34-627010441
† Current address: Department of Infectious Diseases, Hospital Universitario Virgen de las Nieves, Av. de las Fuerzas Armadas nº 2, 18014 Granada, Spain.

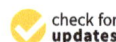

Citation: Hidalgo-Tenorio, C.; Pitto-Robles, I.; Arnés García, D.; de Novales, F.J.M.; Morata, L.; Mendez, R.; de Pablo, O.B.; López de Medrano, V.A.; Lleti, M.S.; Vizcarra, P.; et al. Cefto Real-Life Study: Real-World Data on the Use of Ceftobiprole in a Multicenter Spanish Cohort. *Antibiotics* 2023, 12, 1218. https://doi.org/10.3390/antibiotics12071218

Academic Editor: Mehran Monchi

Received: 19 June 2023
Revised: 14 July 2023
Accepted: 18 July 2023
Published: 21 July 2023

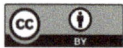

Copyright: © 2023 by the authors. Licensee MDPI, Basel, Switzerland. This article is an open access article distributed under the terms and conditions of the Creative Commons Attribution (CC BY) license (https://creativecommons.org/licenses/by/4.0/).

Abstract: Background: Ceftobiprole is a fifth-generation cephalosporin that has been approved in Europe solely for the treatment of community-acquired and nosocomial pneumonia. The objective was to analyze the use of ceftobiprole medocaril (Cefto-M) in Spanish clinical practice in patients with infections in hospital or outpatient parenteral antimicrobial therapy (OPAT). Methods: This retrospective, observational, multicenter study included patients treated from 1 September 2021 to 31 December 2022. Results: A total of 249 individuals were enrolled, aged 66.6 ± 15.4 years, of whom 59.4% were male with a Charlson index of four (IQR 2–6), 13.7% had COVID-19, and 4.8% were in an intensive care unit (ICU). The most frequent type of infection was respiratory (55.8%), followed by skin and soft tissue infection (21.7%). Cefto-M was administered to 67.9% of the patients as an empirical treatment, in which was administered as monotherapy for 7 days (5–10) in 53.8% of cases. The infection-related mortality was 11.2%. The highest mortality rates were identified for ventilator-associated pneumonia (40%) and infections due to methicillin-resistant *Staphylococcus aureus* (20.8%) and *Pseudomonas aeruginosa* (16.1%). The mortality-related factors were age (OR: 1.1, 95%CI (1.04–1.16)), ICU admission (OR: 42.02, 95%CI (4.49–393.4)), and sepsis/septic shock (OR: 2.94, 95%CI (1.01–8.45)). Conclusions: In real life, Cefto-M is a safe antibiotic, comprising only half of prescriptions for respiratory infections, that is mainly administered as rescue therapy in pluripathological patients with severe infectious diseases.

Keywords: ceftobiprole; sepsis; older; real-world data; OPAT

1. Introduction

There has been a disturbing increase in multi-resistant microorganisms worldwide over the past decade [1], presenting clinicians with major diagnostic and therapeutic challenges. This phenomenon has been associated with a rise in the failure of empirical antibiotic therapies [2] and with a delay before the administration of an effective drug [3], thereby increasing mortality rates [4]. The rate of carbapenemase-resistant *Pseudomonas* spp. is currently >20% in Spain [1], mainly due to efflux pumps and porin losses. Therefore, carbapenem sparing strategies are recommended to attempt to decrease the rate of carbapenemase-producing Enterobacteriaceae. A randomized controlled trial (MERINO) reported a lower mortality rate using meropenem than using piperacillin/tazobactam in patients with ceftriaxone-resistant *Escherichia coli* or *Klebsiella pneumoniae* bloodstream infections. The findings did not support the utilization of piperacillin-tazobactam against these infections [5]. This has fostered the administration of bactericide antibiotics other than piperacillin/tazobactam to treat gram-negative bacteria such as *P. aeruginosa*, including ceftobiprole. Ceftobiprole medocaril (Cefto-M) is a broad-spectrum, fifth-generation cephalosporin against gram-negative cocci and bacilli, ranging from methicillin-resistant *S. aureus* (MRSA) to ampicillin-susceptible *Enterococcus faecalis, faecium*, and *P. aeruginosa*. It is not affected by efflux pumps or porin losses [6]. It has a spectrum of potential interest for the treatment of catheter-related bacteremia, endocarditis, or complicated urine infections. In an experimental study, the bactericide capacity of Cefto-M in biofilm was higher than that of linezolid, vancomycin, or daptomycin against infections caused by MRSA, methicillin-susceptible *S. aureus* (MSSA), or coagulase-negative *staphylococci* (CoNS) [7]. It may, therefore, be useful for treating infections related to devices (intracardiac, cranial leads, etc.), prosthetic valves, endoprostheses, or osteosynthesis materials. It has demonstrated a similar effectiveness to that of other antibiotics in skin and soft tissue infections [8]. Nevertheless, it has only been approved in Europe for the treatment of community-acquired (CAP) and nosocomial (NP) pneumoniae, excluding ventilator-associated pneumonia (VAP).

Clinical trials are the gold standard for approving novel pharmaceutical products or therapies. However, they can differ from actual clinical experience due to their strict eligibility criteria and optimal conditions. Real-world data can help bridge this gap, thereby supporting and accelerating the incorporation of effective new therapies and technologies into routine clinical practices [9]. However, sample sizes have been limited in previous real-life studies on Cefto-M [10]. With this background, this real-life study in Spain was designed to examine the routine administration of Cefto-M in patients with any type of infection in hospital or receiving outpatient parenteral antimicrobial therapy (OPAT), considering the health and safety outcomes and the mortality-related factors.

2. Results

2.1. Cohort Description

The study included 249 individuals with a mean age of 66.6 ± 15.4 years. A total of 59.4% were male and 92.8% were Caucasian with a mean age-adjusted Charlson index of four (IQR 2–6) and 49.4% had cardiovascular risk factors, primarily cardiovascular disease (31.3%), arterial hypertension (29.3%), and diabetes mellitus (28.1%). A total of 20.9% were immunosuppressed, 14.1% had chronic kidney failure, and 11.6% had chronic obstructive pulmonary disease (COPD) (Table 1). The infection origin was nosocomial/healthcare-related in 57% of the patients. Cefto-M was administered in hospital to 95.6% of the patients (80.4% in the medical department) and as OPAT in 4.4% of the patients. Sepsis was present in 26.5%, septic shock in 4.4%, and concomitant COVID-19 infection in 13.7% of the patients. The median number of foci was one (IQR: 1–1). The type of infection was respiratory in 55.8% (CAP in 24.1%, NP in 24.9%, and VAP in 2%); skin and soft tissue infection (SSTI) in

21.7%; and bacteremia in 17.7% of the patients (catheter-related in 2.8% and no focus in 14.9%) (Table 1).

Table 1. Epidemiological characteristics, comorbidities, and infection pathways.

	Cohort N = 249
Age, mean (years), (±SD)	66.6 (±15.4)
Charlson index, median (IQR)	4 (2–6)
Sex, n (%)	
Male	148 (59.4)
Female	101 (40.6)
Ethnicity, n (%)	
Caucasian	231 (92.8)
Latin	17 (6.8)
African	1 (0.4)
Acquisition of the infection, n (%)	
Community-acquired infection	107 (43)
Nosocomial/Nosohusial infection	142 (57)
Presence of sepsis or septic shock, n (%)	
Sepsis	66 (26.5)
Septic shock	11 (4.4)
Inpatient departments, n (%)	238 (95.6)
Medical department	188 (75.5)
Intensive care unit	12 (4.8)
Surgical department	38 (15.2)
Outpatient antibiotic treatment, n (%)	11 (4.4)
Co-infection with SARS-CoV-2 (COVID-19), n (%)	34 (13.7)
Comorbidities	
Cardiovascular risk factors, n (%)	123 (49.4)
Hypertension	73 (29.3)
Dyslipidemia	11 (4.4)
Obesity	1 (0.4)
≥2 Risk factors	38 (15.2)
Cardiovascular disease, n (%)	78 (31.3)
Ischemic heart disease	26 (33.3)
Heart failure	9 (11.5)
Atrial fibrillation/flutter	15 (19.2)
Pacemaker carrier	1 (1.3)
Dilated cardiomyopathy	1 (1.3)
Other conditions	9 (11.5)
≥2 Conditions	17 (21.8)
Respiratory diseases, n (%)	74 (29.7)
Chronic obstructive pulmonary disease (COPD)	29 (39.2)
Obstructive sleep apnea (OSA)	9 (12.2)
Thromboembolic pulmonary vascular disease (TPVD)	4 (5.4)
Bronchiectasis	8 (10.8)
Asthma	4 (5.4)
Interstitial lung disease	3 (4.1)
Other conditions	6 (8.1)
≥2 Conditions	11 (14.9)

Table 1. *Cont.*

	Cohort $N = 249$
Gastrointestinal and hepatic diseases, n (%)	45 (18.1)
Chronic liver disease	18 (40)
Liver cirrhosis	8 (17.8)
Peptic ulcer disease	6 (13.3)
Inflammatory bowel disease	3 (6.7)
Liver transplantation	3 (6.7)
Other conditions	7 (15.6)
Chronic kidney disease, n (%)	35 (14.1)
Active solid malignancy, n (%)	20 (8)
Active hematologic malignancy, n (%)	33 (13.3)
Metabolic disorders, n (%)	83 (33.3)
Diabetes mellitus	70 (84.3)
Hypothyroidism	11 (13.3)
Adrenal insufficiency	2 (2.4)
Neurological diseases, n (%)	21 (8.4)
Stroke, n (%)	14 (5.6)
Psychiatric conditions, n (%)	9 (3.6)
Immunocompromised patients, n (%)	52 (20.9)
Immunosuppressant drugs therapy, n (%)	43 (17.3)
Infection pathway	
Bloodstream infection, n (%)	44 (17.7)
Primary bacteremia	37 (14.9)
Catheter-associated bloodstream infection	7 (2.8)
Infective endocarditis, n (%)	3 (1.2)
Respiratory tract infections, n (%)	139 (55.8)
Nosocomial pneumonia	62 (24.9)
Community-acquired pneumonia	60 (24.1)
Ventilator-associated pneumonia	5 (2)
Soft tissue and skin infection, n (%)	54 (21.7)
Diabetic foot infection	20 (37)
Cellulitis	10 (18.5)
Soft tissue abscess	7 (13)
Infected pressure ulcer	7 (13)
Surgical wound infection	6 (11.1)
Myositis	2 (3.7)
Other type	2 (3.7)
Urinary tract infection, n (%)	10 (4)
Complicated UTI (pyelonephritis)	5 (50)
Non-complicated UTI	3 (30)
Renal abscess	2 (20)
Central nervous system infection, n (%)	8 (3.2)
Ventriculoperitoneal shunt infection	3 (37.5)
Epidural abscess	2 (25)
Cerebral abscess	2 (25)
Meningitis	1 (12.5)
Intra-abdominal infection, n (%)	9 (3.6)

Table 1. Cont.

	Cohort $N = 249$
Bone and joint infection, n (%)	14 (5.6)
Prosthetic joint Infection	6 (42.9)
Osteomyelitis	4 (28.6)
Infectious tenosynovitis	3 (21.4)
Septic arthritis	1 (7.1)
Spondylodiscitis, n (%)	3 (1.2)
Other type of infection, n (%)	4 (1.6)

2.2. Microbiological Isolation

Microbiological isolates were obtained from 137 patients (55%) and were polymicrobial in 56 (40.6%). Among the isolates, 87 (35.3%) were gram-positive cocci (GPC), 20 (22.9%) of which were coagulase-negative staphylococci (CoNS), including 13 (65%) that were methicillin-resistant. A total of 46 (18.4%) were *S. aureus*, including 21 (45.6%) methicillin-susceptible *S. aureus* (MSSA) and 24 (52.3%) methicillin-resistant *S. aureus* (MRSA) isolates. A total of nine (10.3%) were *Enterococcus* spp., including eight (88.9%) *E. faecalis* and one (11.1%) ampicillin-susceptible *E. faecium* isolates. A total of 10 (11.5%) were *Streptococcus* spp., including five (50%) *S. pneumoniae* and five (50%) *Streptococci* of other species. A total of 49 were gram-negative bacilli (GNB), including 13 (26.5%) multi-susceptible *Enterobacteriaceae*, 31 (63.3%) non-fermenting GNB (100% *P. aeruginosa*), and five (10.2%) GNB of other species (*Hemophilus influenzae* [2], *Morganella* spp. [2], and *Moraxella* spp. [1]). Table 2 lists the other variables.

Table 2. Microbial isolates.

	Cohort $N = 249$
General microbial profile, n (%)	
No isolation	111 (45)
Positive microbial samples	137 (55)
Microbial profile of isolates, n (%)	
Monomicrobial infection	81 (59.2)
Polymicrobial infection	56 (40.8)
Gram-positive cocci, n (%)	87 (63.5)
Staphylococus aureus	46 (52.9)
MRSA	24 (52.2)
MSSA	21 (45.6)
Non-categorized *Staphylococcus aureus*	1 (2.2)
CoNS	20 (22.9)
Staphylococcus epidermidis	15 (75)
Staphylococcus hemolyticus	2 (10)
Staphylococcus hominis	2 (10)
Staphylococcus schleiferi	1 (5)
Enterococcus spp.	9 (10.3)
Enterococcus faecalis	8 (88.9)
Enterococcus faecium	1 (11.1)
Streptococcus spp.	10 (11.5)
Streptococcus pneumoniae	5 (50)
Streptococcus anginosus	4 (40)
Streptococcus peroris	1 (10)
Other cocci	2 (2.3)
Rhottia spp.	2 (100)

Table 2. Cont.

	Cohort N = 249
Gram-positive bacilli, n (%)	1 (0.7)
Cutibacterium acnes	1 (100)
Gram-negative bacilli, n (%)	49 (35.8)
Enterobacterales	13 (26.5)
Klebsiella pneumoniae	5 (38.5)
Escherichia coli	4 (30.8)
Klebsiella oxytoca	1 (7.7)
Proteus mirabilis	1 (7.7)
Proteus vulgaris	1 (7.7)
Non-fermenting gram-negative bacilli	31 (63.2)
Pseudomonas aeruginosa	31 (100)
Other gram-negative bacilli	5 (10.2)
Morganella spp.	2 (40)
Hemophilus influenzae	2 (40)
Moraxella catarrhalis	1 (20)

S. aureus: *Staphylococcus aureus*. MRSA: methicillin-resistant *Staphylococcus aureus*. MSSA: methicillin-susceptible *Staphylococcus aureus*. CoNS: coagulase-negative *Staphylococcus* spp.

All the isolated microorganisms treated with Cefto-M were susceptible to this drug (three MRSA, three MSSA, one enterococcus, one streptococcus, and 10 GNB, including four *P. aeruginosa*). Among the GPC, 97.2% (*n* = 35) were susceptible to vancomycin (100% of MRSA, 93.3% of MSSA, and 100% of both enterococci and streptococci). In terms of the GNB susceptibility, 83.3% of the *P. aeruginosa* isolates were susceptible to meropenem, 40% to cefepime, and 70% to piperacillin/tazobactam (Table 3).

Table 3. Susceptibility of microbial isolates.

Microorganisms, n (%)		Vanco-S	Cloxa-S	Dapto-S	Ceftobi-S	Cefe-S	Mero-S	Pip/Taz-S
Staphylococcus aureus	46 (18.4)	35 (97.2)	14 (41.2)	21 (67.7)	6 (100)			
MRSA	24 (9.6)	21 (100)	0 (0)	16 (80)	3 (100)			
MSSA	21 (8.4)	14 (93.3)	14 (100)	5 (45.5)	3 (100)			
Enterococcus spp.	10 (4)	5 (100)	NT	0 (0)	1 (100)			
Streptococcus spp.	10 (4)	3 (100)	NT	NT	1 (100)			
GNB	49 (20.5)				10 (100)	4 (33.3)	5 (83.3)	16 (84.2)
Enterobacteriaceae	13 (5.2)				5 (100)	1 (50)	NT	6 (100)
Pseudomonas aeruginosa	31 (12.4)				4 (100)	2 (40)	5 (83.3)	7 (70)
Hemophilus influenzae	2 (0.4)				1 (100)	1 (100)	NT	NT

GNB: gram-negative bacilli. Vanco-S: vancomycin-susceptible; Cloxa-S: cloxacillin-susceptible; Dapto-S: daptomycin-susceptible; Ceftobi-S: ceftobiprole-susceptible; Cefe-S: cefepime-susceptible; Mero-S: meropenem-susceptible; Pip/Taz-S: piperacillin-tazobactam-susceptible. NT: not tested.

2.3. Outcomes

The median (IQR) stay was 20 (13–32) days. The total Cefto-M dose per patient was 10.5 (7.5–15) g for 7 days (5–10), what was administered in monotherapy to 134 patients (53.8%). It was prescribed as an empirical antibiotic treatment in 67.9% of the patients, and was appropriate in 82.8% of these. It was used as a first-line antibiotic in 74 (29.7%) patients and a second-line or more in 176 (70.3%). It was administered due to the failure of previous antibiotic therapy in 33.7% of the patients and after receiving the microbiology results from 26.1%. The death of 54 patients (21.7%) during the 6-month follow-up was directly attributable to infection in 28 (11.2%) patients, 17 (60.7%) of whom died during the first 14 days, nine (32.1%) between days 15 and 28, and two (7.1%) between day 29 and 6 months. Readmission for the same reason was recorded in 15 patients (6%) and for recurrence during the first month of follow-up in three (1.2%) (Table 4).

Table 4. Outcomes.

	N = 249
Total dose of ceftobiprole, median (IQR)	10.5 (7.5–15)
Duration of antibiotic therapy, median (IQR)	7 (5–10)
Treatment regimen, n (%)	
Ceftobiprole monotherapy	134 (53.8)
Antibiotic combination	115 (46.2)
Ceftobiprole + Daptomycin	27 (23.5)
Ceftobiprole + Vancomycin	4 (3.5)
Ceftobiprole + Linezolid	8 (7)
Ceftobiprole + Dalbavancin	1 (0.9)
Ceftobiprole + Clindamycin	2 (1.7)
Ceftobiprole + Tigecycline	4 (3.5)
Ceftobiprole + Cloxacillin	3 (2.6)
Ceftobiprole + Ceftazidime	1 (0.9)
Ceftobiprole + Ceftaroline	2 (1.7)
Ceftobiprole + Ceftriaxone	2 (1.7)
Ceftobiprole + Ceftazidime/Avibactam	2 (1.7)
Ceftobiprole + Meropenem	9 (7.8)
Ceftobiprole + Levofloxacin	10 (8.7)
Ceftobiprole + Ciprofloxacin	4 (3.5)
Ceftobiprole + Piperacillin/Tazobactam	2 (1.7)
Ceftobiprole + Amikacin	6 (5.2)
Ceftobiprole + Azithromycin	10 (8.7)
Ceftobiprole + Metronidazole	13 (11.3)
Ceftobiprole + Trimethoprim/Sulfamethoxazole	7 (6.1)
Ceftobiprole + Doxycycline	2 (1.7)
Ceftobiprole + Fosfomycin	1 (0.9)
Ceftobiprole + Antifungal agents	6 (5.2)
Ceftobiprole + Antiviral agents	2 (1.7)
Length of hospital stay, median (IQR)	20 (13–32)
Ceftobiprole as empirical treatment, n (%)	169 (67.9)
Appropriate empirical treatment, n (%)	140 (82.8)
Prescription of Ceftobiprole, n (%)	
As first-line treatment	74 (29.7)
As second-line or more	175 (70.3)
Reason for switching to Ceftobiprole, n (%)	
Failure of previous antibiotic treatment	84 (48)
Toxicity/adverse effects of previous antibiotic treatment	3 (1.7)
Guided by microbiological results	65 (37.1)
Other reasons (or combination of previous)	23 (13.1)
Recurrence and readmission, n (%)	
Recurrence of infection (in the first month)	3 (1.2)
Hospital readmission	15 (6)
Mortality, n (%)	
Total mortality	54 (21.7)
Non-related-to-infection mortality	26 (10.4)
Related-to-infection mortality	28 (11.2)
14-day mortality	17 (60.7)
28-day mortality	9 (32.1)
6-month mortality	2 (7.1)

The mortality rate by infection type was 16.7% (10/60) for CAP, 14.5% (9/62) for NP, 40% (2/5) for VAP, 11.4% (5/44) for bacteremia, 5.6% (3/54) for SSTI, and 20% (7/34) for concomitant COVID-19 infection (Figure 1).

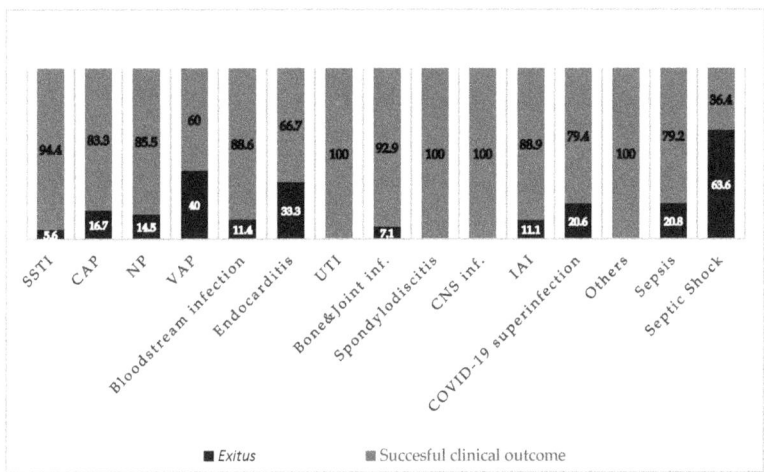

Figure 1. Clinical outcomes by the primary infection type (*n* = 249). SSTI: skin and soft tissue infection; CAP: community-acquired pneumonia; NP: nosocomial pneumonia; VAP: ventilator-associated pneumonia; UTI: urinary tract infection; CNS: central nervous system; IAI: intra-abdominal infection; *Exitus*: death.

The mortality rate was 9.1% (8/88) for infections caused by GPC (MRSA 20.8% [5/24], *E. faecalis* 12.5% [1/8], MSSA 9.5% [2/21], CNS-MR 0% [0/13], *Pneumococcus* 0% [0/5], *E. faecium* S-ampicillin 0% [0/1], *S. pneumoniae* 0% [0/5], and *Streptococcus* spp. 0% [0/5]). The mortality rate was 11.8% (6/51) for infections caused by GNB (*P. aeruginosa* 16.1% [5/31], multi-susceptibility *Enterobacteriaceae* 0% [0/12], and other non-fermenting GNB 0% [0/2]), and 0% in infections by gram-positive bacilli (0/1) (Figure 2).

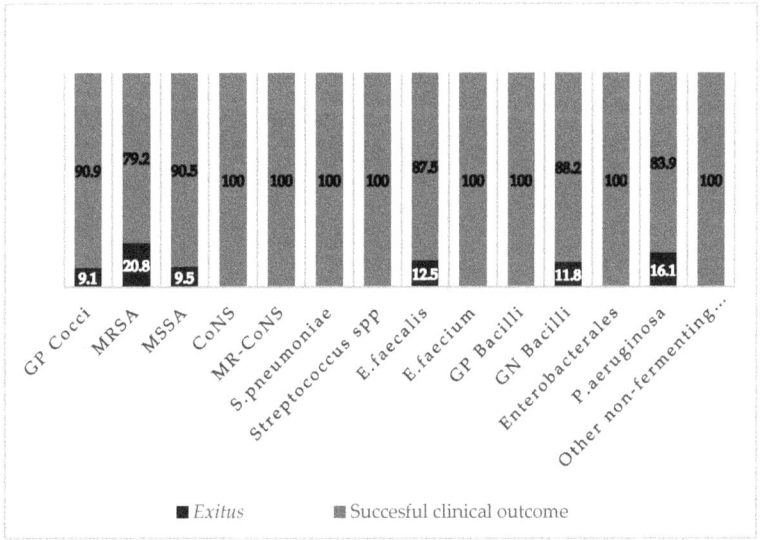

Figure 2. Clinical outcomes of the microbial isolates. GP: gram-positive; MRSA: methicillin-resistant *Staphylococcus aureus*; MSSA: methicillin-susceptible *Staphylococcus aureus*; CoNS: coagulase-negative *Staphylococcus* spp; MR-CoNS: methicillin-resistant coagulase-negative *Staphylococcus* spp; GN: gram-negative; GNB: gram-negative bacilli; *Exitus*: death.

2.4. Adverse Effects

No adverse effect was recorded in 96.4% of the treated patients, a mild effect in 1.6%, and a moderate effect in 1.6%. No patient abandoned the treatment due to adverse effects. Mild hypertransaminasemia was reported in 1.2% of the patients; diarrhea, nausea, and vomiting in 0.8%; and skin rash in 0.4% (Table 5).

Table 5. Adverse drug effects.

	$N = 249$
Total adverse effects, n (%)	9 (3.6)
Severity of adverse effects, n (%)	
Mild	4 (1.6)
Moderate	4 (1.6)
Severe	1 (0.4)
Adverse effects by symptoms, n (%)	
Elevated liver enzymes	3 (1.2)
Gastrointestinal symptoms	2 (0.8)
Urticaria-like cutaneous rash	1 (0.4)

2.5. Bi- and Multivariate Analyses of Mortality-Related Factors

In the bivariate analysis, mortality was associated with higher age (76.7 ± 13.3 vs. 65.3 ± 15.2 yrs.; $p = 0.0001$), ICU admission (28.6 vs. 2.1%; $p = 0.001$), cardiovascular risk factors (78.6 vs. 45.7%, $p = 0.001$), underlying neurological disease (21.4 vs. 6.8%; $p = 0.019$), immunodepression (35.7 vs. 19%; $p = 0.04$), sepsis/septic shock (57.1 vs. 27.6%; $p = 0.0001$), VAP (7.1 vs. 1.4%, $p = 0.04$), fewer days of Cefto-M treatment (six [P25–P75: 3–8.5] vs. seven [P25–P75: 5–10] days, $p = 0.029$), and a lower total dose (in mg) of Cefto-M (nine [4.5–12.75] vs. 10.5 [7.5–15], $p = 0.049$). Hospitalization in a department/unit of infectious diseases emerged as a protective factor (24.9% vs. 7.1%; $p = 0.035$).

In the multivariate analysis, the factors associated with infection-related mortality were age (OR: 1.1 95% CI [1.04–1.16]), sepsis/septic shock (OR 2.94, 95% CI [1.01–8.54]), and ICU admission (OR 42.02, 95% CI [4.49–393.4]) (Table 6).

Table 6. Mortality risk factors: bivariate and multivariate analyses.

	Non-Survivor $N = 31$	Survivor $N = 219$	Bivariate p *	Multivariate HR, 95% IC
Age (±DS)	76.7 (±13.3)	65.3 (±15.2)	0.0001	1.1 (1.04–1.16)
Charlson index, mean (IQR)	4.5 (4–6.75)	4 (2–6)	0.253	
Sex, n (%)				
Men	20 (71.4)	128 (57.9)	0.17	
Women	8 (28.6)	93 (44.1)		
Ethnicity, n (%)				
Caucasian	27 (96.4)	204 (92.3)		
Latin	1 (3.6)	16 (7.2)	0.718	
African	0 (0)	1 (0.5)		
Inpatient department, n (%)	26 (83.9)	212 (95.9)	0.9	
Medical services	24 (92.3)	167 (78.8)		
Infectious diseases	2 (7.1)	55 (24.9)	0.035	0.19 (0.03–1.2)
Internal medicine	9 (32.1)	43 (19.5)	0.12	
Pneumology	2 (7.1)	37 (16.7)	0.27	
Intensive care unit	8 (28.6)	4 (1.8)	0.001	42.02 (4.49–393.4)
Hematology	1 (3.6)	10 (4.5)	0.25	
Oncology	2 (7.1)	14 (6.3)	0.27	
Surgical services	2 (7.1)	36 (16.3)	0.27	
OPAT, n (%)	2 (7.1)	9 (4.1)	0.36	

Table 6. Cont.

	Non-Survivor N = 31	Survivor N = 219	Bivariate p*	Multivariate HR, 95% IC
Comorbidities, n (%)				
Cardiovascular risk factors	22 (78.6)	101 (45.7)	0.001	1.67 (0.49–5.62)
Cardiovascular disease	6 (21.4)	72 (32.6)	0.231	
Pulmonary disease	10 (35.7)	64 (29)	0.461	
Gastrointestinal and hepatic disease	5 (17.9)	40 (18.1)	0.975	
Chronic kidney disease	4 (14.3)	31 (14)	0.97	0.94 (0.21–4.33)
Active solid malignancy	3 (10.7)	17 (7.7)	0.526	1.81 (0.289–11.41)
Hematological malignancy	4 (14.3)	29 (13.1)	0.864	1.21 (0.24–6.16)
Metabolic disorders	11 (39.3)	72 (32.6)	0.478	
Neurological diseases	6 (21.4)	15 (6.8)	0.019	2.59 (0.69–9.85)
Psychiatric disorders	0 (0)	9 (4.1)	0.6	
Stroke	3 (10.7)	11 (5)	0.199	
Immunosuppression	10 (35.7)	42 (19)	0.04	2.03 (0.52–7.88)
COVID-19 superinfection, n (%)	7 (25)	27 (12.2)	0.063	2.08 (0.43–10.12)
Number of pathway infection, mean (IQR)	1 (1–1)	1 (1–1)	0.945	
Pathway infection, n (%)				
Bloodstream infection	5 (17.9)	39 (17.6)	0.978	
Infective endocarditis	1 (3.6)	2 (0.9)	0.223	
Communitary-acquired pneumonia	10 (35.7)	50 (22.6)	0.127	
Nosocomial pneumonia	9 (32.1)	53 (24)	0.347	
Ventilator-associated pneumonia	2 (7.1)	3 (1.4)	0.04	0.12 (0.004–3.89)
Skin and soft tissue infection	3 (10.7)	51 (23.1)	0.135	
Urinary tract infection	0 (0)	10 (4.5)	0.251	
Central nervous system infection	0 (0)	8 (3.6)	0.306	
Intra-abdominal infection	1 (3.6)	8 (3.6)	0.99	
Bone and joint infection	1 (3.6)	13 (5.9)	0.617	
Spondylodiscitis	0 (0)	3 (1.4)	0.535	
Other type of infection	0 (0)	4 (1.8)	0.473	
Sepsis or shock	16 (57.1)	61 (27.6)	0.0001	2.94 (1.01–8.54)
Microbiology and acquisition of the infection, n (%)				
Microbial isolation			0.758	
Monomicrobial infection	9 (32.1)	84 (38)		
Polymicrobial infection	6 (21.4)	50 (22.6)		
Place of acquisition of the infection			0.762	
Communitary-acquired infection	12 (42.9)	95 (43)		
Nosocomial infection	10 (35.7)	90 (40.7)		
Nosohusial infection	6 (21.4)	36 (16.4)		
GPC	8 (28.6)	80 (36.2)	0.426	
MRSA	5 (17.9)	19 (8.6)	0.118	
MSSA	2 (7.1)	19 (8.6)	0.794	
CoNS	0 (0)	20 (9)	0.097	
Enterococcus faecalis	1 (3.6)	7 (3.2)	0.909	
Streptococcus pneumoniae	0 (0)	5 (2.3)	0.421	
GNB	6 (21.4)	45 (20.4)	0.895	
Pseudomonas aeruginosa	5 (17.9)	26 (11.8)	0.358	

Table 6. Cont.

	Non-Survivor N = 31	Survivor N = 219	Bivariate p *	Multivariate HR, 95% IC
Antimicrobial therapy				
Total dose of ceftobiprole (mg), mean (IQR)	9 (4.5–12.75)	10.5 (7.5–15)	0.049	0.91 (0.73–1.12)
Length of ceftobiprole therapy (days), mean (IQR)	6 (3–8.5)	7 (5–10)	0.029	1.08 (0.82–1.4)
Therapy regimen:				
Ceftobiprole monotherapy, n (%)	16 (57.1)	118 (53.4)	0.708	
Antibiotic combination, n (%)	12 (42.9)	103 (46.6)		
Prescription of ceftobiprole:				
First-line, n (%)	6 (21.4)	68 (30.8)	0.308	1.34 (0.4–4.49)
Rescue therapy, n (%)	22 (78.6)	153 (69.2)		
Empirical treatment, n (%)	22 (78.6)	146 (66.1)	0.183	

OPAT: outpatient parenteral antibiotic therapy; GPC: gram-positive cocci; CoNS: coagulase-negative staphylococcus; GNB: gram-negative bacilli; MRSA: methicillin-resistant *Staphylococcus aureus*; MSSA: methicillin-susceptible *S. aureus*. HR: hazard ratio, 95% CI: 95% confidence interval. * $p < 0.05$ as significant.

3. Discussion

The patients in this real-life study were elderly, largely male, and pluripathological, with a high comorbidity index and a predominance of cardiovascular risk factors. Around one in five were immunodepressed, one in seven had kidney failure, and one in ten had COPD. More than half of the infections were nosocomial or healthcare-related, and approx. 5% received OPAT. As in the case of other beta-lactams, the pharmacokinetics and pharmacodynamics of Cefto-M favor its infusion for 24 h, making it a potentially useful antibiotic for OPAT regimens in the patients with infections caused by GPC, including MRSA and ampicillin-susceptible *Enterococcus* spp., and by non-ESLB-producing GNB such as *Pseudomonas* spp. [11].

More than one-third of the participants had sepsis/septic shock, and one-seventh were co-infected with SARS-CoV-2 (COVID-19). Septic shock was described as an independent mortality risk factor with an increase in the risk of up to 12% for every hour in shock, regardless of the focus, isolate, type of poly/monomicrobial infection, or presence/absence of bacteremia [12]. A multicenter study of more than 5000 individuals with septic shock reported a mortality rate of approx. 50% when the antibiotic treatment was appropriate and 89% when it was not [13]. Co-infection with SARS-CoV-2 in critical patients with NP or VAP has been known to worsen the prognosis, although it does not increase the rate of invasive fungal infection or change the type of microorganism isolated at respiratory level [14]. In the present study, only approx. half of the patients received Cefto-M for respiratory infections (half NP and half CAP), which is the sole indication for this antibiotic in Spain [15]. One-fifth of the patients were treated for skin/soft tissue infections and one-sixth for bacteremia. Cefto-M was effective against *Enterococcus* in a murine model of a UTI [16] and was proposed as a possible treatment for a complicated UTI produced by *Pseudomonas* spp. [17]. Three non-inferiority clinical trials in the patients with skin and soft tissue infections reported no difference between Cefto-M and its comparators in terms of clinical or microbiological responses or safety profiles [18]. The decisions of clinicians to prescribe Cefto-M to the remaining patients in this real-life study were supported by pharmacokinetic [19] and in vitro [20] studies. In addition, Cefto-M was used to treat gram-negative bacterial (GNB) infections to avoid the utilization of carbapenems and help reduce the incidence of carbapenemase-producing *Enterobacteriaceae*. Furthermore, in the cases of infection caused by methicillin-resistant CGP such as MRSA, which were all susceptible to vancomycin, Cefto-M was prescribed instead of this lipoglycopeptide due to its rapid bactericidal activity, high volume of distribution to tissues, and excellent safety profile. Only two real-life studies have been published on this issue, one with only 51 patients [10] and a recent study [21] with a smaller sample size (n = 198) than in the present investigation (n = 249).

The total crude infection-related mortality in these patients was 11.2%, most frequently due to VAP (40%), followed by pneumonia with COVID-19 co-infection (20%), CAP requiring hospitalization (16.7%), NP (14.5%), bacteremia (11.4%), and skin/soft tissue infections (5.6%). Among the microorganisms, the highest mortality rates were for MRSA (20.8%) and *P. aeruginosa* (16.1%). The mortality rate was <1% in the clinical trials of Cefto-M in the patients with CAP. The difference between the present findings might be explained by their stricter eligibility criteria, with the exclusion of the patients receiving an antibiotic for >24 h in the previous three days and those with aspiration pneumonia, viral respiratory infections, polymicrobial infections, or radiological or clinical suspicions of atypical pneumonia [22]. In the trial for the patients with NP, the total mortality rate was 16.7% and the infection-attribution rate was 5.9%. This major discrepancy with the present findings can again be attributed to the trial eligibility criteria, which excluded the patients receiving systemic antibiotic treatment for >24 h in the previous two days and those with severe kidney failure or liver failure, evidence of infection with ceftazidime- or Cefto-M-resistant pathogens, and clinical circumstances potentially hampering the evaluation of the effectiveness, e.g., sustained shock, active tuberculosis, pulmonary abscess, or post-obstructive pneumonia [23].

Only one patient (0.4%) had a severe complication. However, the treatment was not withdrawn from any patient due to an adverse effect, similar to the findings of a single-center real-life study on the use of Cefto-M in 29 patients with infections in a third-level hospital [24].

Finally, the main factors related to mortality in this cohort of Cefto-M-treated patients were older age (the mean age of the patients was 76.7 years), the presence of sepsis/septic shock, and ICU admission, which have all been independently related to higher infection-related mortality rates in the previous studies [25].

The study was limited by its retrospective design and possible selection bias. Its strengths included its multicenter design, sample size (largest to date), and real-life nature, reflecting as faithfully as possible the utilization of Ceftobiprole-M in routine clinical practices in Spain.

4. Materials and Methods

4.1. Study Design

This real-life, retrospective, multicenter, observational, and descriptive study on the use of Cefto-M included patients in hospital or receiving OPAT with nosocomial/nosohusial or community-acquired infections from 12 Spanish centers in six autonomous communities (Andalusia, Madrid, Cataluña, Valencia, Murcia, and Cantabria). The study period was from the time of the drug's approval in 2021 to 31 December 2022. The study was approved by the Provincial Ethics Committee of Granada (ref: 0095-N-22), with no requirement for the informed consent of the patients. All the data were gathered in accordance with the Spanish personal data protection legislation (Organic Law 3/5 December 2018) and the Declaration of Helsinki.

This descriptive study did not involve a pharmacological intervention. The treatments were always prescribed by the attending physicians according to their clinical practice.

The inclusion criteria was as follows: age > 17 years; receipt of Cefto-M as the first-line or rescue treatment for $\geq$48 h ($\geq$six vials in the patients with normal renal function, creatinine clearance-adjusted in the patients with kidney failure); and $\geq$30 days of follow-up post-discharge or, in the case of the patients with osteomyelitis o endocarditis, $\geq$6 months post-discharge.

The exclusion criteria was as follows: pregnancy, allergy to beta-lactams, or any formulation excipient.

4.2. Variables and Definitions

The variables of this study included the following: age, sex, ethnicity, days of hospitalization (dates of admission and discharge), prescribing hospital department, age-adjusted Charlson index, and comorbidities.

The infection types in this study included the following: bacteremia (complicated/non-complicated], endocarditis (definite/probable/suspected, native/early prosthetic/late prosthetic/on pacemaker), respiratory infection (upper tract/CAP/NP/VAP), urinary tract infection (UTI), central nervous system infection, spondylodiscitis, osteoarticular infection, intra-abdominal infection, or other foci of infection. The etiology of the infections in this study included the following: community or nosocomial/nosohusial/healthcare-related; sepsis or septic shock, monomicrobial/polymicrobial infection, and co-infection with SARS-CoV-2 (COVID-19).

In this study, Cefto-M was administration as monotherapy or combination therapy (for the same infection); empirical or targeted administration; first-line or rescue (due to poor response to previous antibiotherapy, microbiology results, or toxicity with previous antibiotherapy), and was based on the days of administration, dose, and adverse events.

Previous antibiotic (for same infection) with treatment duration.

The microbiology for this study consisted of the microorganism causing the infection and the antibiogram according to the EUCAST criteria [26]. The EUCAST cutoff points were as follows for: *Staphylococci* (Vancomycin (*S. aureus*): 2; Vancomycin (CoNS): 4; Oxacillin (*S. aureus*): 2; Oxacillin (CoNS): 0.25); *Enterococci* (Vancomycin: 4); *Pneumococci* (Cefepime: 1; Ceftobiprole: 0.5; Vancomycin: 2; Meropenem: 2); *Enterobacteriaceae* (Cefepime: 1; Ceftobiprole: 0.25; Meropenem: 2); and *Pseudomonas aeruginosas* (Cefepime: 0.001; Ceftobiprole: insufficient evidence; Meropenem: 2).

Infection-related mortality at 14 and 28 days (at 6 months for endocarditis or osteomyelitis); readmission for the same reason during the first month; and relapse/recurrence of the infection.

The definitions of the terms used in this study are as follows.

- Nosocomial infection: onset > 72 h after hospitalization.
- Nosohusial/nosocomial infection: healthcare-related (day hospital, residence, day center for elderly).
- The age-adjusted Charlson comorbidity index was used to estimate the 10-year life expectancy of the patients as a function of their age and the presence of comorbidities at admission for the infectious episode [27].
- Sepsis/septic shock: refractory hypotension and end-organ perfusion dysfunction despite adequate fluid resuscitation [28].
- Immunodepression: congenital or acquired immunodeficiency or receipt of immunosuppressive treatment [29].
- Relapse/recurrence of the infection was defined by a second episode within three months [30].
- The adverse effect classification used in this study is as follows.
    - Mild: required no antidote or treatment; brief hospitalization.
    - Moderate: required treatment modification (e.g., dose adjustment, combination with another drug) but no interruption of drug administration. A longer hospitalization or prescription of a specific treatment may be needed.
    - Severe: threatened the life of the patient and mandated an interruption of the drug administration and prescription of a specific treatment.
    - Lethal: directly or indirectly contributed to the death of a patient.

4.3. Sample Size

A sample size of approx. 250 individuals was estimated to be adequate to analyze the use of Cefto-M in routine clinical practices with a confidence interval of 95% and an error of 5%. The information was obtained from the electronic records of the different hospital pharmacy departments, gathering the number of patients to whom the drug was administered based on the type of infection. These data were introduced into an anonymized database in an SPSS format, following the national data protection legislation and the principles of the Declaration of Helsinki.

4.4. Statistical Analysis

In a descriptive analysis, the absolute and relative frequencies (%) were calculated for the qualitative variables. The means with standard deviation were calculated for the quantitative variables with a normal distribution and the medians were4 calculated with an interquartile range (IQR) for the variables with a non-normal distribution (Kolmogorov–Smirnov test).

In the bivariate analyses of the mortality-related factors, the chi-squared test was used to compare the qualitative variables, the Student's *t*-test was used for the quantitative variables a with normal distribution, and the Mann–Whitney U test for those with non-normal distribution. A multivariate logistic regression analysis considered the variables that were statistically significant in a bivariate analysis or deemed relevant (i.e., chronic kidney failure, active hematological or solid organ neoplasia, co-infection by SARS-CoV-2, rescue/first-line treatment).

Ethics approval and consent to participate: This study was approved by the ethics committee of the coordinating center and was exempted from the need to obtain informed consent due to its retrospective design and large size. All the data were gathered in accordance with Spanish personal data protection legislation.

5. Conclusions

Ceftobiprole-M is a safe antibiotic, comprising only half of the prescriptions for patients with respiratory infection, that is mainly administered as rescue therapy in pluripathological patients with severe infections. The infection-related mortality was 11.2%, which was largely associated with higher age, the presence of sepsis/septic shock, and ICU admission.

Author Contributions: Conceptualization, C.H.-T.; methodology, C.H.-T.; software, I.P.-R., F.J.M.d.N., L.M., R.M., O.B.d.P., V.A.L.d.M., M.S.L., P.V., J.L.-T., A.A.G., L.M.N., M.M. and M.P.R.S.; formal analysis, C.H.-T. and I.P.-R.; validation, I.P.-R., F.J.M.d.N., L.M., R.M., O.B.d.P., V.A.L.d.M., M.S.L., P.V., J.L.-T., A.A.G., L.M.N., M.M. and M.P.R.S.; formal analysis, C.H.-T., I.P.-R. and D.A.G.; investigation, C.H.-T., I.P.-R. and D.A.G.; resources, I.P.-R. and D.A.G.; data curation, I.P.-R. and D.A.G.; writing—original draft preparation, C.H.-T.; writing—review and editing, I.P.-R. and S.S.-D.; visualization, F.J.M.d.N., L.M., R.M., O.B.d.P., V.A.L.d.M., M.S.L., P.V., J.L.-T., A.A.G., L.M.N., M.M. and M.P.R.S.; supervision, S.S.-D.; project administration, C.H.-T. and I.P.-R.; funding acquisition, C.H.-T. All authors have read and agreed to the published version of the manuscript.

Funding: The Project received partial funding from the laboratory ADVANZ PHARMA Switzerland, at 2 rue de Jargonnant, 5th floor, 1207 Geneva, Switzerland. FIB-CEF-2021-01.

Institutional Review Board Statement: The study was conducted in accordance with the Declaration of Helsinki and approved by the Ethics Committee of Granada (CEIM/CEI of Granada); code: 0095-N-22.

Informed Consent Statement: This study was exempt from the need to obtain patient consent due to its retrospective design and large size.

Data Availability Statement: The researchers confirm the accuracy and availability of the data used in this study.

Conflicts of Interest: The authors declare no conflict of interest. The funders had no role in the design of the study; in the collection, analyses, or interpretation of the data; in the writing of the manuscript; or in the decision to publish the results.

References

1. Annual Surveillance Reports on Antimicrobial Resistance. EARS-Net. For 2019. Available online: https://antibiotic.ecdc.europa.eu/en (accessed on 1 May 2023).
2. Kollef, M.H. Inadequate antimicrobial treatment: An important determinant of outcome for hospitalized patients. *Clin. Infect. Dis.* **2000**, *31* (Suppl. 4), S131–S138. [CrossRef] [PubMed]
3. Funk, D.J.; Parrillo, J.E.; Kumar, A. Sepsis and septic shock: A history. *Crit. Care Clin.* **2009**, *25*, 83–101. [CrossRef] [PubMed]
4. Micek, S.T.; Hampton, N.; Kollef, M. Risk Factors and Outcomes for Ineffective Empiric Treatment of Sepsis Caused by Gram-Negative Pathogens: Stratification by Onset of Infection. *Antimicrob. Agents Chemother.* **2017**, *62*, e01577-17. [CrossRef]
5. Harris, P.N.A.; Tambyah, P.A.; Lye, D.C.; Mo, Y.; Lee, T.H.; Yilmaz, M.; Alenazi, T.H.; Arabi, Y.; Falcone, M.; Bassetti, M.; et al. Effect of Piperacillin-Tazobactam vs Meropenem on 30-Day Mortality for Patients with E coli or Klebsiella pneumoniae Bloodstream Infection and Ceftriaxone Resistance: A Randomized Clinical Trial. *JAMA* **2018**, *320*, 984–994. [CrossRef]
6. Del Pozo, J.L.; Patel, R. Ceftobiprole medocaril: A new generation beta-lactam. *Drugs Today* **2008**, *44*, 801–825. [CrossRef]
7. Abbanat, D.; Shang, W.; Amsler, K.; Santoro, C.; Baum, E.; Crespo-Carbone, S.; Lynch, A.S. Evaluation of the in vitro activities of ceftobiprole and comparators in staphylococcal colony or microtitre plate biofilm assays. *Int. J. Antimicrob. Agents* **2014**, *43*, 32–39. [CrossRef] [PubMed]
8. Noel, G.J.; Strauss, R.S.; Amsler, K.; Heep, M.; Pypstra, R.; Solomkin, J.S. Results of a double-blind, randomized trial of ceftobiprole treatment of complicated skin and skin structure infections caused by gram-positive bacteria. *Antimicrob. Agents Chemother.* **2008**, *52*, 37–44. [CrossRef]
9. Berger, M.L.; Sox, H.; Willke, R.J.; Brixner, D.L.; Eichler, H.G.; Goettsch, W.; Madigan, D.; Makady, A.; Schneeweiss, S.; Tarricone, R.; et al. Good practices for real-world data studies of treatment and/or comparative effectiveness: Recommendations from the joint ISPOR-ISPESpecial Task Force on real-world evidence in health care decision making. *Pharmacoepidemiol. Drug Saf.* **2017**, *26*, 1033–1039. [CrossRef]
10. Zhanel, G.G.; Kosar, J.; Baxter, M.; Dhami, R.; Borgia, S.; Irfan, N.; MacDonald, K.S.; Dow, G.; Lagacé-Wiens, P.; Dube, M.; et al. Real-life experience with ceftobiprole in Canada: Results from the CLEAR (CanadianLEadership onAntimicrobialReal-life usage) registry. *J. Glob. Antimicrob. Resist.* **2021**, *24*, 335–339. [CrossRef]
11. López-Cortés, L.E.; Herrera-Hidalgo, L.; Almadana, V.; Gil-Navarro, M.V.; DOMUS OPAT Group. Ceftobiprole, a new option for multidrug resistant microorganisms in the outpatient antimicrobial therapy setting. *Enferm. Infecc. Microbiol. Clin.* **2022**, *40*, 399–400. [CrossRef]
12. Kumar, A.; Roberts, D.; Wood, K.E.; Light, B.; Parrillo, J.E.; Sharma, S.; Suppes, R.; Feinstein, D.; Zanotti, S.; Taiberg, L.; et al. Duration of hypotension before initiation of effective antimicrobial therapy is the critical determinant of survival in human septic shock. *Crit. Care Med.* **2006**, *34*, 1589–1596. [CrossRef]
13. Kumar, A.; Ellis, P.; Arabi, Y.; Roberts, D.; Light, B.; Parrillo, J.E.; Dodek, P.; Wood, G.; Kumar, A.; Simon, D.; et al. Initiation of inappropriate antimicrobial therapy results in a fivefold reduction of survival in human septic shock. Antimicrobial Therapy of Septic Shock Database Research Group. *Chest* **2009**, *136*, 1237–1248. [CrossRef] [PubMed]
14. Rouzé, A.; Martin-Loeches, I.; Povoa, P.; Makris, D.; Artigas, A.; Bouchereau, M.; Lambiotte, F.; Metzelard, M.; Cuchet, P.; Geronimi, C.B.; et al. Relationship between SARS-CoV-2 infection and the incidence of ventilator-associated lower respiratory tract infections: A European multicenter cohort study. *Intensive Care Med.* **2021**, *47*, 188–198. [CrossRef] [PubMed]
15. Agencia Española de Medicamentos y Productos Sanitarios. CIMA. Ministerio de Sanidad. Gobierno de España. Available online: https://cima.aemps.es/cima/publico/home.html (accessed on 1 May 2023).
16. Singh, K.V.; Murray, B.E. Efficacy of ceftobiprole Medocaril against *Enterococcus faecalis* in a murine urinary tract infection model. *Antimicrob. Agents Chemother.* **2012**, *56*, 3457–3460. [CrossRef] [PubMed]
17. Bassetti, M. Strategies for management of difficult to treat Gram-negative infections: Focus on *Pseudomonas aeruginosa*. *Infez. Med.* **2007**, *15*, 20–26. [PubMed]
18. Lan, S.H.; Lee, H.Z.; Lai, C.C.; Chang, S.P.; Lu, L.C.; Hung, S.H.; Lin, W.-T. Clinical efficacy and safety of ceftobiprole in the treatment of acute bacterial skin and skin structure infection: A systematic review and meta-analysis of randomized controlled trials. *Expert Rev. Anti-Infect. Ther.* **2022**, *20*, 95–102. [CrossRef] [PubMed]
19. Barbour, A.; Schmidt, S.; Rout, W.R.; Ben-David, K.; Burkhardt, O.; Derendorf, H. Soft-tissue penetration of ceftobiprole in healthy volunteers determined by in vivo microdialysis. *Antimicrob. Agents Chemother.* **2009**, *53*, 2773–2776. [CrossRef]
20. Yin, L.Y.; Calhoun, J.H.; Thomas, J.K.; Shapiro, S.; Schmitt-Hoffmann, A. Efficacies of ceftobiprole medocaril and comparators in a rabbit model of osteomyelitis due to methicillin-resistant *Staphylococcus aureus*. *Antimicrob. Agents Chemother.* **2008**, *52*, 1618–1622. [CrossRef]
21. Gentile, I.; Buonomo, A.R.; Corcione, S.; Paradiso, L.; Giacobbe, D.R.; Bavaro, D.F.; Tiseo, G.; Sordella, F.; Bartoletti, M.; Palmiero, G.; et al. CEFTO-CURE study: CEFTObiprole Clinical Use in Real-lifE-a multi-centre experience in Italy. *Int. J. Antimicrob. Agents* **2023**, *62*, 106817. [CrossRef]
22. Nicholson, S.C.; Welte, T.; File, T.M., Jr.; Strauss, R.S.; Michiels, B.; Kaul, P.; Balis, D.; Arbit, D.; Amsler, K.; Noel, G.J. A randomised, double-blind trial comparing ceftobiprole medocaril with ceftriaxone with or without linezolid for the treatment of patients with community-acquired pneumonia requiring hospitalisation. *Int. J. Antimicrob. Agents* **2012**, *39*, 240–246. [CrossRef]

23. Awad, S.S.; Rodriguez, A.H.; Chuang, Y.C.; Marjanek, Z.; Pareigis, A.J.; Reis, G.; Scheeren, T.W.L.; Sánchez, A.S.; Zhou, X.; Saulay, M.; et al. A phase 3 randomized double-blind comparison of ceftobiprole medocaril versus ceftazidime plus linezolid for the treatment of hospital-acquired pneumonia. *Clin. Infect. Dis.* **2014**, *59*, 51–61. [CrossRef] [PubMed]
24. Durante-Mangoni, E.; Andini, R.; Mazza, M.C.; Sangiovanni, F.; Bertolino, L.; Ursi, M.P.; Paradiso, L.; Karruli, A.; Esposito, C.; Murino, P.; et al. Real-life experience with ceftobiprole in a tertiary-care hospital. *J. Glob. Antimicrob. Resist.* **2020**, *22*, 386–390. [CrossRef] [PubMed]
25. Taylor, E.H.; Marson, E.J.; Elhadi, M.; Macleod, K.D.M.; Yu, Y.C.; Davids, R.; Boden, R.; Overmeyer, R.C.; Ramakrishnan, R.; Thomson, D.A.; et al. Factors associated with mortality in patients with COVID-19 admitted to intensive care: A systematic review and meta-analysis. *Anaesthesia* **2021**, *76*, 1224–1232. [CrossRef] [PubMed]
26. The European Committee on Antimicrobial Susceptibility Testing. Breakpoint Tables for Interpretation of MICs and Zone Diameters. Version 13.0. 2023. Available online: http://www.eucast.org (accessed on 1 May 2023).
27. Charlson, M.E.; Charlson, R.E.; Paterson, J.C.; Marinopoulos, S.S.; Briggs, W.M.; Hollenberg, J.P. The Charlson comorbidity index is adapted to predict costs of chronic disease in primary care patients. *J. Clin. Epidemiol.* **2008**, *61*, 1234–1240. [CrossRef]
28. Cecconi, M.; Evans, L.; Levy, M.; Rhodes, A. Sepsis and septic shock. *Lancet* **2018**, *392*, 75–87. [CrossRef]
29. Ramirez, J.A.; Musher, D.M.; Evans, S.E.; Dela Cruz, C.; Crothers, K.A.; Hage, C.A.; Aliberti, S.; Anzueto, A.; Arancibia, F.; Arnold, F.; et al. Treatment of Community-Acquired Pneumonia in Immunocompromised Adults: A Consensus Statement Regarding Initial Strategies. *Chest* **2020**, *158*, 1896–1911. [CrossRef]
30. Miguel Cisneros-Herreros, J.; Cobo-Reinoso, J.; Pujol-Rojo, M.; Rodríguez-Baño, J.; Salavert-Lletí, M. Guía para el diagnóstico y tratamiento del paciente con bacteriemia. Guías de la Sociedad Española de Enfermedades Infecciosas y Microbiología Clínica (SEIMC). *Enfermedades Infecc. Microbiol. Clin.* **2007**, *25*, 111–130. [CrossRef]

Disclaimer/Publisher's Note: The statements, opinions and data contained in all publications are solely those of the individual author(s) and contributor(s) and not of MDPI and/or the editor(s). MDPI and/or the editor(s) disclaim responsibility for any injury to people or property resulting from any ideas, methods, instructions or products referred to in the content.

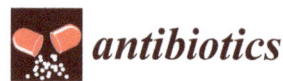

Article

Antimicrobial Stewardship in COVID-19 Patients: Those Who Sow Will Reap Even through Hard Times

Marcella Sibani [1,*], Lorenzo Maria Canziani [2], Chiara Tonolli [3], Maddalena Armellini [2], Elena Carrara [2], Fulvia Mazzaferri [1], Michela Conti [2], SAVE Working Group [†], Annarita Mazzariol [4], Claudio Micheletto [5], Andrea Dalbeni [6], Domenico Girelli [7] and Evelina Tacconelli [2]

1. Infectious Diseases Department, Azienda Ospedaliera Universitaria Integrata Verona, 37126 Verona, Italy
2. Division of Infectious Diseases, Department of Diagnostics and Public Health, University of Verona, 37129 Verona, Italy
3. Department of Pharmacy, Azienda Ospedaliera Universitaria Integrata Verona, 37126 Verona, Italy
4. Microbiology and Virology Section, Department of Diagnostic and Public Health, University of Verona, 37129 Verona, Italy
5. Respiratory Unit, Cardio-Thoracic Department, Azienda Ospedaliera Universitaria Integrata Verona, 37126 Verona, Italy
6. Section General Medicine C and Liver Unit, Department of Medicine, Azienda Ospedaliera Universitaria Integrata Verona, 37126 Verona, Italy
7. Department of Medicine, Section of Internal Medicine D, University of Verona, 37129 Verona, Italy
* Correspondence: marcella.sibani@aovr.veneto.it
† Collaborators: SAVE working group: Cinzia Arena, Lorenzo Barbato, Fabiana Busti, Alessandra Consolaro, Paola del Bravo, Laura Maccacaro, Anna Mantovani, Pietro Minuz, Maria Diletta Pezzani, Giulia Sartori.

Citation: Sibani, M.; Canziani, L.M.; Tonolli, C.; Armellini, M.; Carrara, E.; Mazzaferri, F.; Conti, M.; SAVE Working Group; Mazzariol, A.; Micheletto, C.; et al. Antimicrobial Stewardship in COVID-19 Patients: Those Who Sow Will Reap Even through Hard Times. *Antibiotics* **2023**, *12*, 1009. https://doi.org/10.3390/antibiotics12061009

Academic Editors: Gyöngyvér Soós and Ria Benkő

Received: 13 May 2023
Revised: 29 May 2023
Accepted: 1 June 2023
Published: 4 June 2023

Copyright: © 2023 by the authors. Licensee MDPI, Basel, Switzerland. This article is an open access article distributed under the terms and conditions of the Creative Commons Attribution (CC BY) license (https://creativecommons.org/licenses/by/4.0/).

Abstract: Background: Since the SARS-CoV-2 pandemic emerged, antimicrobial stewardship (AS) activities need to be diverted into COVID-19 management. Methods: In order to assess the impact of COVID-19 on AS activities, we analyzed changes in antibiotic consumption in moderate-to-severe COVID-19 patients admitted to four units in a tertiary-care hospital across three COVID-19 waves. The AS program was introduced at the hospital in 2018. During the first wave, COVID-19 forced the complete withdrawal of hospital AS activities. In the second wave, antibiotic guidance calibration for COVID-19 patients was implemented in all units, with enhanced stewardship activities in Units 1, 2, and 3 (intervention units). In a controlled before and after study, antimicrobial usage during the three waves of the COVID-19 pandemic was compared to the 12-month prepandemic unit (Unit 4 acted as the control). Antibiotic consumption data were analyzed as the overall consumption, stratified by the World Health Organization AWaRe classification, and expressed as defined-daily-dose (DDD) and days-of-therapy (DOT) per 1000 patient-day (PD). Results: In the first wave, the overall normalized DOT in units 2–4 significantly exceeded the 2019 level (2019: 587 DOT/1000 PD ± 42.6; Unit 2: 836 ± 77.1; Unit 3: 684 ± 122.3; Unit 4: 872, ± 162.6; $p < 0.05$). After the introduction of AS activities, consumption decreased in the intervention units to a significantly lower level when compared to 2019 (Unit 1: 498 DOT/1000 PD ± 49; Unit 2: 232 ± 95.7; Unit 3: 382 ± 96.9; $p < 0.05$). Antimicrobial stewardship activities resulted in a decreased amount of total antibiotic consumption over time and positively affected the watch class and piperacillin-tazobactam use in the involved units. Conclusions: During a pandemic, the implementation of calibrated AS activities represents a sound investment in avoiding inappropriate antibiotic therapy.

Keywords: COVID-19; antimicrobial stewardship; antibiotic consumption

1. Introduction

The pandemic caused by the severe acute respiratory syndrome coronavirus 2 (SARS-CoV-2) has deeply impacted countless aspects of the national healthcare system. Among others, the inappropriate use of antimicrobial agents, especially during the first phase of the pandemic, raised special concern in terms of antibiotic stewardship (AS) [1] and the possible spread of multidrug-resistant (MDR) bacteria [2]. Several authors report an increase in antibiotic consumption, particularly during the first months of the COVID-19 pandemic, with respect to pre-COVID-19 times [3–10].

Although several guidance documents for antibiotic usage have been developed to recommend against routine usage of antibiotics in this population [11,12], the estimated proportion of COVID-19 patients receiving antibiotic therapy is close to 60% [1,13]. Several factors have been recognized as potential drivers of antibiotic overprescription: reduction of AS activities due to personnel reallocation, decreased screening for MDR organisms, shortage of specific antibiotics, difficulty in diagnosis of coinfections, and rapid turn-over of personnel [14–16]. However, there is evidence reporting a very low rate of bacterial coinfections in patients with SARS-CoV-2 infection. In a meta-analysis reviewing data up to April 2020, Langford et al. [17] and Lansbury et al. [18] found a rate ranging between 4 and 6% of patients and up to 14% of healthcare-associated infections in critically ill patients in intensive care units (ICU) [19]. Similarly, in a recent meta-analysis including studies up to May 2021, the prevalence of confirmed bacterial coinfection was 4% in the overall population and 12% in critically ill patients [1].

To tackle the misuse of antibiotics, various strategies have been proposed. However, clear recommendations on AS in a pandemic or in infectious diseases with pandemic potential have not been developed due to limited evidence [4,20–23].

Our work aims to substantially add to the existing evidence by evaluating the impact of a multiphase and customized AS intervention in non-ICU COVID-19 wards during the first three waves of the COVID-19 pandemic.

2. Results

Overall, the intervention included 1743 patients and 29,112 PD.

2.1. Antimicrobial Consumption

Nearly 40,000 individual drug administrations were analyzed. During the first pandemic wave (March–June 2020), overall consumption largely exceeded the desirable consumption estimate of 587 days of therapy (DOT)/1000 patient days (PD) (95% C.I. 559.4–613.7) (based on the levels of consumption achieved after prepandemic AS intervention [24]) for all the units (Unit 2: 836, 95% C.I. 143.0–1528; Unit 3: 684, 95% C.I. 489–878.1; Unit 4: 872, 95% C.I. 468.1–1275.9), but Unit 1, which was the last to be activated in April. Figure 1 shows the overall anatomical therapeutic chemical classification system (ATC) J01 antimicrobial consumption across the study period compared to the prepandemic consumption level.

After the intervention, consumption reduced in all the wards. Consumption in Units 1–3 significantly reduced compared to the 2019 level, while in Unit 4 overall consumption data fell in the referral range. The annual whole-hospital antimicrobial consumption expressed by defined daily dose (DDD)/1000 PD was of 715, 811, and 732 in 2019, 2020, and 2021, respectively. Table 1 summarized the mean overall consumption per wave and per unit, compared to the referral consumption level.

Overall normalized antimicrobial consumption as expressed by DOT showed a significant and progressive decrease across the three waves for Unit 1 (−29 DOT/1000 PD, −5.5%), Unit 2 (−604 DOT/1000 PDs, −72%), and Unit 3 (−302 DOT/1000 PDs, −44%), while no significant variation emerged for Unit 4 (control Unit). For Units 2 and 3, significant reductions over time occurred also for DDD, length of therapy (LOT), and World Health Organization (WHO) watch class antimicrobials. Detailed data are provided in Table 2. Antibiotic consumption according to WHO AwaRe classes is shown in Figure 2.

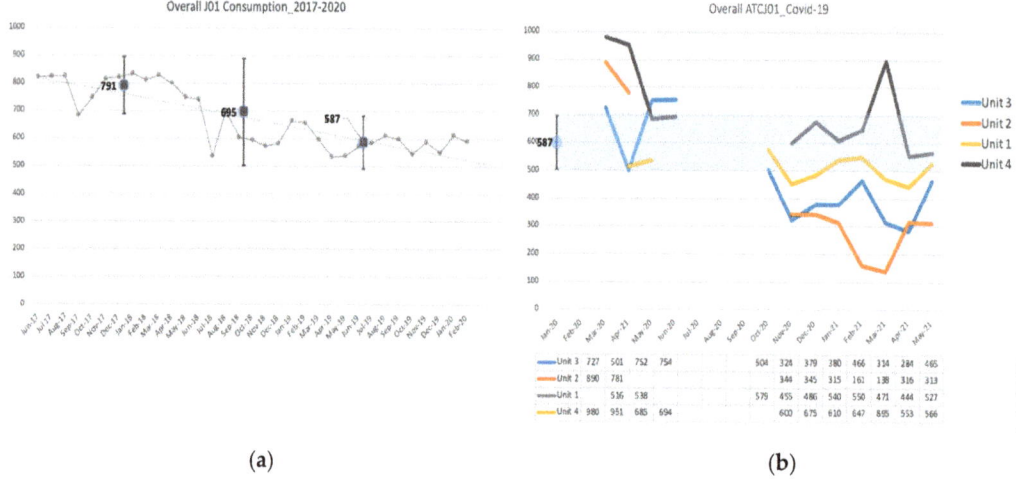

(a)　　　　　　　　　　　　　　　　　(b)

Figure 1. Comparison of the overall ATC-J01 antimicrobial consumption in the prepandemic period and during the COVID-19 pandemic: (**a**) Consumption trend (DOT/1000 PD) in the hospital's medical area targeted by the hospital's AS program in the period 2017–2019 [24]; (**b**) consumption trends (DOT/1000 PD) in the 4 COVID-19 dedicated wards; monthly consumption data in the COVID-19 period are provided in the table.

Table 1. Comparison of the overall antimicrobial consumption (DOT/1000 PD) to the desirable consumption estimate for the Medical Area [21].

		Antimicrobial Consumption (ATC J01) DOT/1000 PD					
Unit	Medical Area Desirable Consumption Estimate Mean (SD)	Wave 1 Mean (SD)	*p*-Value *	Wave 2 Mean (SD)	*p*-Value *	Wave 3 Mean (SD)	*p*-Value *
Unit 1 (WHO Scale 5)		527 (±15.6)	0.082	515 (±55.3)	**0.0168**	498 (±49)	**0.0037**
Unit 2 (WHO Scale 3–4)	587 (±42.6)	836 (±77.1)	**<0.001**	335 (±17.0)	**<0.001**	232 (±95.7)	**<0.001**
Unit 3 (WHO Scale 4)		684 (±122.3)	**0.027**	397 (±76.1)	**<0.001**	382 (±96.9)	**<0.001**
Unit 4 (C) (WHO Scale 4–5)		872 (±162.6)	**<0.0001**	628 (±40.7)	0.1496	665 (±159)	0.1236

* Student's T test; C = control. WHO Scale = World Health Organization Ordinal Scale for clinical improvement in COVID-19 patients: 1: ambulatory patients, no limitation of activities; 2: ambulatory patients, with limitation of activities; 3: hospitalized patients, no oxygen therapy needed; 4: hospitalized patients, oxygen by mask or nasal cannulae needed; 5: hospitalized, severe disease, noninvasive ventilation, or high flow oxygen needed.

When consumptions were stratified according to WHO AWaRe classes [25], we observed substantial variation between units for watch antimicrobials: Unit 4 showed higher consumption when compared to all the other wards in both waves two and three; the difference in the amount of employed piperacillin-tazobactam had a similar trend, accounting for 30–50% of the total watch variation. Amoxicillin-clavulanate was the most prescribed antibiotic from the access class in all four wards and in all periods, accounting for 68%, 82%, 49%, and 63% of total access consumption in Units 1, 2, 3, and 4, respectively. Considering watch class, piperacillin/tazobactam accounted for one-third of the consumption (32–44%), followed by ceftriaxone (20–27%) and meropenem (7–15%). In the reserve class, linezolid was the most commonly used agent (36–58%), followed by new cephalosporins/beta-lactamase inhibitors (11–32%) and daptomycin (9–31%).

Table 2. Comparison of antimicrobial consumption data across waves and units.

Outcome	Unit	First Wave Mean (DS)	Second Wave Mean (DS)	Third Wave Mean (DS)	p-Value *
DOT/1000 PD	Unit 1	527 (±15.6)	515 (±55.3)	498 (±49)	<0.05
	Unit 2	836 (±77.1)	334.7 (±17.0)	232 (±95.7)	<0.05
	Unit 3	684 (±122.3)	397 (±76.1)	382 (±96.9)	<0.05
	Unit 4(C)	872 (±162.6)	628 (±40.7)	665 (±159)	>0.05
DDD/1000 PD	Unit 1	635 (±217.1)	575 (±94.2)	533 (±80.9)	>0.05
	Unit 2	913 (±137.9)	319(±34)	219 (±96.3)	<0.05
	Unit 3	736 (±150.4)	408 (±67.9)	430 (±111.7)	<0.05
	Unit 4(C)	834 (±209.8)	576 (±42.7)	636 (±183.0)	data
LOT/1000 PD	Unit 1	407 (±43.8)	444 (±49.0)	411(±38.6)	>0.05
	Unit 2	614 (±36.1)	294 (±15)	201 (±74.4)	<0.05
	Unit 3	524 (±73.5)	327 (±55.1)	307 (±69.7)	<0.05
	Unit 4(C)	702 (±95.6)	532 (±50.7)	514 (±102.8)	data
ACCESS (DOT/1000 PDs)	Unit 1	57 (±26.2)	101 (±23.6)	107.5 (±8.2)	>0.05
	Unit 2	157 (±31.8)	67 (±16.1)	52 (±47.9)	>0.05
	Unit 3	155 (±91.7)	84 (±35.1)	109 (±34.7)	>0.05
	Unit 4(C)	194 (±71.4)	60 (±29.5)	111 (±41.3)	>0.05
WATCH (DOT/1000 PDs)	Unit 1	369(±101.8)	379 (±61.5)	338.8 (±33.9)	>0.05
	Unit 2	640 (±72.2)	243 (±26.9)	172 (67.7)	<0.05
	Unit 3	456 (±83)	277 (±38.8)	245 (56.5)	<0.05
	Unit 4(C)	632 (±103.3)	513 (±116.6)	472 (82.3)	>0.05
RESERVE (DOT/1000 PDs)	Unit 1	101 (±91.2)	35 (±35.1)	52 (±13.9)	>0.05
	Unit 2	39 (±26.9)	25 (±14.4)	9 (±10.3)	>0.05
	Unit 3	72 (±9.9)	36 (±12.3)	29 (±22.0)	>0.05
	Unit 4(C)	46 (±22.9)	56 (±70.4)	81 (49.3)	>0.05
PIPERACILLIN-TAZOBACTAM (DOT/1000 PDs)	Unit 1	93 (±55.2)	112 (±37.7)	143 (±49.6)	>0.05
	Unit 2	161 (±43.8)	124 (±15.5)	73.2 (±16.4)	<0.05
	Unit 3	142 (±63.6)	114 (±23.6)	103 (±29.9)	<0.05
	Unit 4(C)	276 (±32.8)	225 (±34.6)	212 (±39.0)	<0.05

* ANOVA test for repeated measures; C = control.

2.2. Microbiological and Clinical Outcomes

Positive blood cultures were detected in 7% of patients and were stable over time for each unit (ranging 3–10% in individual wards). Multidrug-resistant bacteria were etiological agents in 2.7% of positive blood cultures, ranging from 1.1 to 4.0% according to the unit. C. difficile infections were stable over the waves and compared with the prepandemic period (23 cases in total, 0.8 cases/100 admitted patients, <1.5/1000 PD for every period analyzed). No clusters were detected. No significant difference in microbiological outcomes emerged when analyzed within or between the three units across time.

The mean mortality rate across all three periods was 16%; it was higher for Units 1 and 4. When analyzed over the three waves, no significant variation emerged for any ward. The mean length of stay (LOS) was 7 ± 2, 7 ± 1.5, and 8 ± 3 days in the three waves, respectively. No significant variation intra- or interunits could be identified.

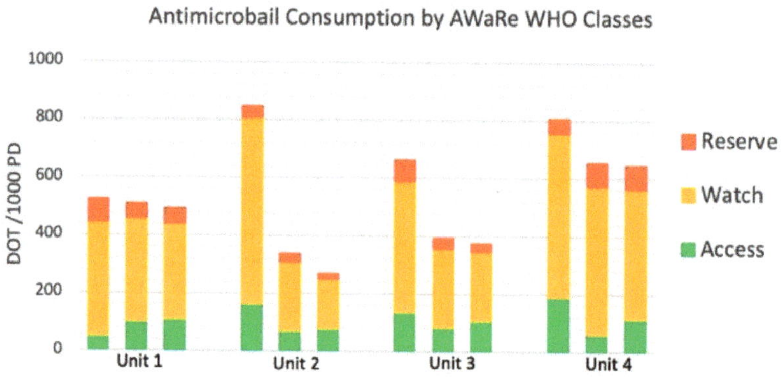

Wave	1	2	3	1	2	3	1	2	3	1	2	3
Access	9%	19%	22%	19%	20%	28%	20%	21%	28%	23%	9%	17%
Watch	76%	71%	68%	77%	72%	66%	69%	70%	64%	71%	78%	70%
Reserve	14%	9%	10%	4%	8%	6%	11%	9%	7%	6%	12%	12%

Figure 2. Normalized DOT/1000 PD of AWaRe antibiotics; overall consumption is reported as the percentage of access, watch, and reserve by COVID-19 waves.

2.3. *Qualitative Indicators*

During the third wave (February–May 2021), 22 prospective audits were conducted in the three units involved in AS activities, with 503 individual patient charts being reviewed. The prevalences of patients receiving any antibiotic therapy on the audit day in Units 1, 2, and 3 were, respectively, 37%, 22%, and 24%. The overall prescribing appropriateness ranging 67–74%. Targeted therapies accounted for 33–52% of the total prescription, with a mean appropriateness of 78%.

3. Discussion

Several authors reported increasing antibiotic consumption in the first months of the pandemic when compared to previous years and were early advocates of the AS principles being applied and promoted even in this difficult situation [21]. Despite this, very few AS studies were implemented in real-life COVID-19 patients. In this study, we showed that an AS intervention calibrated for COVID-19 patients can control the risk of increased inappropriate antibiotic therapy during a pandemic. Antimicrobial consumption in all wards peaked in wave 1, exceeding the pre-pandemic consumption level in Units 2–4. After AS intervention implementation, consumption tends to reduce, but significant variation across the waves was observed only for Units 1–3 involved in the enhanced AS intervention, where lower WHO watch antimicrobial consumption also occurred.

Published studies of antibiotic use during the COVID-19 pandemic mainly report aggregate whole-hospital normalized antibiotic consumption [9,23,26,27] rather than assessing specifically COVID-19 dedicated wards [28]. The whole-hospital consumption increase has been reported up to 10–15% when compared to the prepandemic period [26,28]; in our facility, we observed a +13% increase in the whole-hospital overall antibiotic consumption (DDD/1000 PD) between 2019 and 2020, while focusing on the COVID-19 wards in the first wave, the variation was between −10% and +48% (mean + 24%). Our reported level of absolute consumption in the first wave was close to the one of 700.3 (±354.8) DDD/1000 occupied bed days (OBD) reported by Guisado-Gil et al. in a tertiary-care hospital in Spain during the first COVID-19 wave [28]. Most of the studies also underline that the higher level of consumption observed during the first months of the pandemic [4,20,22] was followed by a sharp reduction after the immediate introduction of the simple AS bundle [22,29]. Y Liew et al. [20] recorded an increase in defined daily dose (DDD)/100 patient-days (PD) in the first months of 2020 vs. 2019 (54 vs. 47); nonetheless, by the third month into the pandemic, DDD/100 bed day gradually declined to settle at levels similar to the previous year. A. Murgadella-Sancho et al. [4] noted that the mean consumption of antibiotics during hospitalization was lower in 2020 than in 2019 (57.8 DDD/100 PD vs. 64.7 DDD/100 PD), except for March 2020 (80 DDD/100 PD). M. Staub et al. [22] observed weekly duration of therapy (DOT)/1000 PD in medical and ICU wards: the former experienced an increase of 145.3 DOT/1000 PD initially, followed by a decline (362 DOT/1000 PD) after implementation of a bundle of AS interventions; the latter experienced an initial rise of 204, then a reduction of 226.3 DOT/10000 PD.

In our study, analyzing the decreasing consumption trend over subsequent COVID-19 waves, significant variation was identified only in the wards where enhanced AS activities were implemented. The comparisons of DOT and LOT levels and trends for each ward provide some useful insight: in both Units 2 and 3, the decrease in DOT between waves 1 and 2 largely overcomes the reduction in LOT, thus reflecting not only a reduction in duration of therapy or prevalence of patients receiving antibiotics but also a substantial reduction in combination therapies; the DOT to LOT differences of the last two waves are pretty much closer, suggesting the further reduction in this last phase resulted from a reduced start or duration of antibiotic course. In Unit 1, no significant reduction in LOT emerged, suggesting that the reduction of combination therapies played a major role in the overall reduction. The prevalence of patients receiving any antibiotic treatment as recorded by audits performed in Units 1–3 during the third wave was below 40%, thus substantially lower than reported in the first COVID-19 months [1,13] but in line with the literature focusing on later pandemic phases [30].

Different patients' case-mix (especially in terms of clinical severity and comorbidities) and the level of care provided certainly strongly influenced the total consumption level observed in each ward as well as the composition in terms of AwaRe classes. Units 2 and 3 admitted patients with lower clinical severity (WHO 3–4 severity index); prescribers in these units were also the most trained in AS. Since the very beginning of wave 2, antibiotic use has dramatically dropped and tended to stabilize at a level lower than expected in the medical area. This low consumption probably reflects a judicious antibiotic use in the COVID-19 moderately severe patients' population, where a very low rate of coinfection and hospital-acquired infections occurred. This was also confirmed by the high prescribing appropriateness registered by audits. Units 1 and 4, on the contrary, cared mostly for patients with a more severe presentation (WHO 5 severity index) and patients from the ICU after clinical improvement. A higher rate of consumption could be forecast for this setting. Interestingly, despite higher personnel and patient turn-over and bed capacity, Unit 1 showed a substantially lower overall, watch class, and piperacillin/tazobactam consumption when compared to Unit 4. Unit 1 total normalized DOT was significantly lower than expected in waves 2 and 3; piperacillin/tazobactam level was the lowest consumption in wave 1 and showed the lowest mean across the whole 12-month period, thus preventing a significant trend from emerging. In Unit 4, on the contrary, although decreasing, the piperacillin-tazobactam DOT level represents the highest among the four wards in all the waves, thus suggesting further room to curb wide-spectrum antibiotic overprescribing.

The significant reduction or stability of Watch antimicrobials in the context of reducing consumption led to a favorable shift in the AWaRe relative composition of consumption, as shown in Figure 2, with the access representing close to 30% and the watch not reaching 70% of the total consumption in units involved in AS initiatives. Reserve antimicrobial prescription, as for hospital policy, was restricted to infectious disease consultants, and limited to target treatment of MDR-caused infections or specific indications based on the Italian Medicine Agency requirement, thus, we did not regard them as a target for our AS initiative.

Even accounting for different patients' case-mixes and other possible biases, an association between AS activities and improved antibiotic use, both in quantitative and qualitative terms, emerged from these considerations. Different baseline prescribing skills, restricted resource availability and limited time availability suggested personalized AS activities for each ward: a baseline, early, and diffuse intervention was aimed at increasing antibiotic guidelines usability through the dissemination of a mobile and web-based app; then periodical infectious disease (ID)-attendance to clinical rounds was introduced, prioritising resources based on the context complexity and previous AS training; finally, prospective audits were introduced to further focus on and ensure improvement not only in the amount but primarily in the quality of prescriptions.

Bloodstream infections were uncommon and stable over time; *C. difficile* infections were rare, and no clusters were detected. These observations appear to be in line with the literature [17,26]. COVID-19 mortality was deeply entwined with the epidemic phase, demographics, clinical presentation, and standard of care [31]. In our study, the crude in-hospital mortality rate varied widely with unit and wave, with the higher rate observed in units admitting more severe patients and providing higher intensity of care; overall mortality rate of 16%, which is in line with published reports for in-hospital mortality [32–34]. No data suggested that reduced antibiotic use was associated with increased mortality, thus confirming the safety of the intervention.

Strengths and Limitations

There are several strengths to this study. Most importantly, our AS intervention consisted of simple and highly replicable actions: the introduction of internal guidelines, the attendance of clinical rounds by an ID specialist, and the use of prospective audits. Moreover, the process and the results of this intervention were evaluated using different indicators, belonging to different domains, such as appropriateness of description through audit, antimicrobial consumption summarized from prescription-level data, and microbiological and clinical outcomes. Data were systematically collected through the hospital data repository for the whole study period. Selected metrics of antibiotic consumption were robust within each other and showed similar levels of consumption to independent evaluations through audits.

This study is not without limitations. The full-time allocation of 1 ID specialist represented the most resource-consuming aspect of this intervention, limiting its feasibility, especially in small hospitals. Specific to our setting, time-varying biases due to the pandemic's continuously changing landscape limited the results' generalizability. These biases may be represented, for example, by changes in clinical practice, the case mix of patients, and personnel turnover. In a rapidly evolving situation such as COVID-19, it remains difficult to measure treatment effects, especially in the AS setting. The inconstant activation of COVID-19 wards based on the extremely variable rate of hospitalization made data collection time points intermittent and disjointed, thus preventing us from performing interrupted time series analysis as generally recommended to evaluate AS initiative effectiveness. [35]. Microbiological outcomes were not tailored to the COVID-19 pandemic: samples from the respiratory tract could have represented a better estimate of the incidence of bacterial co-infection. The common pitfalls of AS studies that are present in our study are the use of surrogate measures (e.g., rate of positive blood cultures representing infection rate) and the use of aggregated data that limits the statistical approach.

4. Materials and Methods

A controlled before-and-after study was conducted in a 1350-bed tertiary care, university hospital in Verona, Italy, from March 2020 to May 2021. For the purpose of the study and data analysis, the COVID-19 pandemic was stratified in 3 waves: March–June 2020; October 2020–January 2021; and February–May 2021.

Antimicrobial consumption in the COVID-19 wards was first compared to pre-COVID-19 consumption data. Using the published data from the SAVE AS intervention [24], we assumed that the normalized antibiotic consumption captured in the AS intervention follow-up in 2019 would represent the desirable antimicrobial consumption for the medical wards in our hospital.

The whole hospital's annual antimicrobial consumption data from 2019–2021 was also calculated to identify general trends and provide a benchmark.

Then, we analyzed the antimicrobial consumption in the study wards across the three pandemic waves to evaluate whether any variation occurred before and after the implementation of an enhanced, COVID-19-calibrated AS intervention in 3 wards; another COVID-19 ward, not involved in the enhanced AS activities, served as a control.

4.1. Setting

The study includes 4 units reserved for COVID-19 patients not requiring mechanical ventilation: Unit 1 had a bed capacity ranging from 15 to nearly 50 and a 16-bed semi-intensive section for patients requiring noninvasive ventilation (NIV) or high-flow nasal cannula (HNFC) (WHO Ordinal Scale for clinical improvement level 5); Unit 2 admitted both severe and moderate patients and was used as a "step-down" ward for post-acute patients (WHO outcome scale 3–4) with a bed capacity increasing from 20 to 42; Unit 3 had 34-bed and provided standard care (low-flow oxygen to HNFC but no NIV), treating predominantly severe COVID-19 patients (WHO Severity score 4); and Unit 4 admitted subcritical and post-ICU patients with a bed capacity ranging from 10 to 20, selected as control unit. The period of activity and patient days (PD) for each ward across the three main pandemic waves occurring in our geographical area are shown in Figure 3.

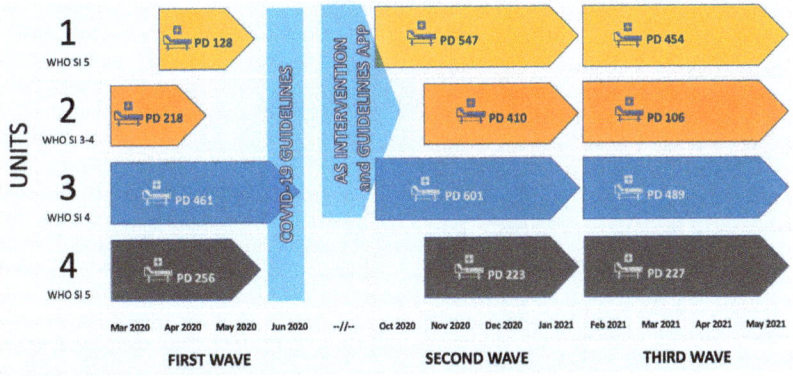

Figure 3. AS intervention timeline and patient days (PD) per unit per wave. *WHO SI = World Health Organization Ordinal Scale for clinical improvement in COVID-19 patients: 1: ambulatory patients, no limitation of activities; 2: ambulatory patients, with limitation of activities; 3: hospitalized patients, no oxygen therapy needed; 4: hospitalized patients, oxygen by mask or nasal cannulae needed; 5: hospitalized, severe disease, noninvasive ventilation, or high flow oxygen needed.

4.2. Intervention

The University Hospital of Verona implemented an AS team in 2018. In the same year, a comprehensive AS intervention was implemented in 4 hospital medical wards and achieved a significant reduction in antimicrobial consumption sustained beyond the intervention's completion in the 21-month post-intervention period. During 2019, consumption in the included wards stabilized with a mean value of 587 DOT/1000 PDs (95% C.I. 559.4–613.7). As extensive audits simultaneously detected high prescribing appropriateness, we assumed this level would represent a fair estimate of the desired consumption level in the specific context of the local medical area [24].

During the first COVID-19 wave, AS activities were interrupted as the AS teams were fully dedicated to COVID-19 management. Formal internal guidelines addressing COVID-19 treatment and antibiotic management in COVID-19 patients were disseminated in all 4 units at the end of the first wave. No antibiotic treatment was routinely recommended for COVID-19 patients, regardless of clinical severity. The guidelines limited antibiotic therapy for those patients presenting with clinical, laboratory, or radiological data, suggesting bacterial coinfection; in that case, referral to the already existing hospital guidelines for empiric antibiotic treatment was advised. ID consultations were available upon request for all the non-ID-led units.

In the second wave, AS interventions were progressively re-established and calibrated on the COVID-19 patients, with diversified enhanced activities in Units 1–3:

- Since October 2020, an ID specialist has attended daily Unit 1 clinical rounds to support antibiotic prescription and withholding and advise on the diagnostic process. Biweekly revision of ongoing antibiotic therapies was also resumed in Unit 2, already involved in the pre-COVID-19 AS intervention, to refresh physicians' diagnostic and prescribing skills.
- Starting from the third wave, the COVID-19 guidelines as well as the hospital antibiotic guidelines were made available through the Firstline app, available for iOS and Android, and on the web (https://firstline.org/, accessed on 28 April 2023) for Units 1–3, to increase their usability; local epidemiological data and monographs of antibiotics were also accessible from the same platform.
- Prospective audits were conducted weekly in the three intervention units during the third wave. All the patients receiving antibiotic therapy on the audit day had their electronic health records reviewed; quality indicators such as compliance with empirical therapy guidelines and appropriateness of therapy were evaluated and recorded.

The intervention timeline is shown in Figure 3.

4.3. Outcomes

The primary outcome was the overall antibiotic consumption measured as defined daily dose (DDD), days of therapy (DOT), and length of therapy (LOT) and normalized per 1000 patient days (PD). Defined daily dose is defined as the assumed average maintenance dose per day for a drug used for its main indication in adults, which was calculated according to the WHO ATC Index [36]. DOT is defined as the aggregate sum of days for which any amount of a specific antimicrobial agent was administered to an individual patient (i.e., if a patient receives more than one antibiotic, more than one DOT per day would be counted), while LOT represents the number of days that a patient receives systemic antimicrobial agents, irrespective of the number of different antibiotics [37].

For the 4 units, included in the study, antimicrobial consumption data encompassing all the ATCJ01 drugs administered to patients were retrieved from the hospital's electronic prescribing system. Whole-hospital consumption data were retrieved by the pharmacy's annual report based on the drug dispensing database.

As secondary outcomes, we analyzed:

- consumption data broken down to a single agent and stratified by WHO AWaRe classification (access, watch, reserve) [25].
- prescribing appropriateness as registered by prospective audits. All the patients receiving antibiotic therapy on the audit day had their clinical charts reviewed for presumptive infective diagnosis, antimicrobial prescription, and microbiological results. Appropriateness of therapy was defined as compliance with antibiotic guidelines for empirical therapy and as adequate coverage plus de-escalation if needed for targeted, microbiological-based, therapy. The prevalence of patients receiving antibiotics on the audit day was also collected.
- Clinical outcomes, including in-hospital mortality (measured as crude rate in-hospital mortality) and length of stay (LOS).
- microbiological outcomes, including total bloodstream infection (BSI), BSI caused by MDR bacteria (i.e., methicillin-resistant *S. aureus* and *S. epidermidis*, carbapenem-resistant Enterobacterales and *P. aeruginosa*, ESBL-producing gram-negative, vancomycin-resistant Enterococci, and *C. difficile* infections (incidence per 100 admitted patients, deduplication was applied, counting only the first isolates/positive tests per patient in a 28-day interval, common contaminants were manually removed).

All the outcomes were measured monthly.

4.4. Statistical Analysis

Descriptive statistics were used for antibiotic consumption.

A Student's *t*-test was employed to compare the individual unit overall antimicrobial consumption in each of the three subsequent COVID-19 waves to the 2019 mean consumption. Variation in consumption within each ward across the three periods was appraised using an ANOVA for repeated measures. A *p*-value less than 0.05 was regarded as significant. The analysis was carried out using STATA software (© StataCorp LLC, College Station, TX, USA).

5. Conclusions

Even in a challenging context such as a pandemic, attentively allocating resources to retain AS programs in place represents a sound investment in order to preserve the quality of care and the patient's safety. Essential enabling AS activities can be readapted to effectively face the emerging need even in a resource-constrained setting to ensure that the essential level of prescribing appropriateness is met.

Author Contributions: Conceptualization, E.C., M.S. and E.T.; methodology, M.S. and E.C.; formal analysis, M.S., L.M.C. and C.T.; investigation, L.M.C., M.S., E.C., F.M., M.C., D.G., A.D., C.M. and the SAVE Working Group; data curation, L.M.C.; writing—original draft preparation, M.S., L.M.C., M.A. and A.M.; writing—review and editing, E.C. and E.T.; visualization, M.S. and L.M.C.; project administration, E.C.; funding acquisition, E.T. All authors have read and agreed to the published version of the manuscript.

Funding: This research was funded as a part of the ENSURE study, by the COMBACTE MAG-NET EPI-Net project. EPI-Net receives financial support from the Innovative Medicines Initiative Joint Undertaking under grant agreement No. 115737, the resources of which are composed of financial contributions from the European Union Seventh Framework Programme (FP7/2007-2013) and the European Federation of Pharmaceutical Industries and Association (EFPIA) companies' in-kind contributions.

Institutional Review Board Statement: The study was conducted in accordance with the Declaration of Helsinki and approved by the local Ethics Committee of Azienda Ospedaliera Universitaria Integrata di Verona on 21 December 2020 (protocol code 69359).

Informed Consent Statement: All the data have been collected while maintaining confidentiality in accordance with national data legislation. Patient consent was waived in accordance with the Verona University Hospital's ethical regulations due to the study being considered a quality improvement initiative rather than an experimental study.

Data Availability Statement: The data presented in this study and not contained within the article are available upon request from the corresponding author. The data are not publicly available due to hospital ethical policies.

Acknowledgments: Successful AS activity implementation would not be possible without the precious cooperation of all the healthcare staff caring for COVID-19 patients at our hospital during the challenging and prolonged pandemic and the support of the whole institution. The authors would like to thank all the clinicians, nurses, and supportive personnel at the Azienda Ospedaliera Universitaria Integrata of Verona for their shared effort to provide high-quality care through troublesome times.

Conflicts of Interest: The authors declare no conflict of interest.

References

1. Calderon, M.; Gysin, G.; Gujjar, A.; McMaster, A.; King, L.; Comandé, D.; Hunter, E.; Payne, B. Bacterial co-infection and antibiotic stewardship in patients with COVID-19: A systematic review and meta-analysis. *BMC Infect. Dis.* **2023**, *23*, 14. [CrossRef]
2. Langford, B.J.; Soucy, J.-P.R.; Leung, V.; So, M.; Kwan, A.T.; Portnoff, J.S.; Bertagnolio, S.; Raybardhan, S.; MacFadden, D.R.; Daneman, N. Antibiotic resistance associated with the COVID-19 pandemic: A systematic review and meta-analysis. *Clin. Microbiol. Infect.* **2023**, *29*, 302–309. [CrossRef]
3. Grau, S.; Hernández, S.; Echeverría-Esnal, D.; Almendral, A.; Ferrer, R.; Limón, E.; Horcajada, J.P.; Catalan Infection Control and Antimicrobial Stewardship Program (VINCat-PROA). Antimicrobial Consumption among 66 Acute Care Hospitals in Catalonia: Impact of the COVID-19 Pandemic. *Antibiotics* **2021**, *10*, 943. [CrossRef]

4. Murgadella-Sancho, A.; Coloma-Conde, A.; Oriol-Bermúdez, I. Impact of the strategies implemented by an antimicrobial stewardship program on the antibiotic consumption in the coronavirus disease 2019 (COVID-19) pandemic. *Infect. Control. Hosp. Epidemiol.* **2022**, *43*, 1292–1293. [CrossRef]
5. Vaughn, V.M.; Gandhi, T.N.; Petty, L.A.; Patel, P.K.; Prescott, H.C.; Malani, A.N.; Ratz, D.; McLaughlin, E.; Chopra, V.; Flanders, S.A. Empiric Antibacterial Therapy and Community-onset Bacterial Coinfection in Patients Hospitalized With Coronavirus Disease 2019 (COVID-19): A Multi-hospital Cohort Study. *Clin. Infect. Dis.* **2021**, *72*, e533–e541. [CrossRef]
6. Karami, Z.; Knoop, B.T.; Dofferhoff, A.S.M.; Blaauw, M.J.T.; Janssen, N.A.; van Apeldoorn, M.; Kerckhoffs, A.P.M.; van de Maat, J.S.; Hoogerwerf, J.J.; Oever, J.T. Few bacterial co-infections but frequent empiric antibiotic use in the early phase of hospitalized patients with COVID-19: Results from a multicentre retrospective cohort study in The Netherlands. *Infect. Dis.* **2021**, *53*, 102–110. [CrossRef]
7. Van Laethem, J.; Wuyts, S.; Van Laere, S.; Koulalis, J.; Colman, M.; Moretti, M.; Seyler, L.; De Waele, E.; Pierard, D.; Lacor, P.; et al. Antibiotic prescriptions in the context of suspected bacterial respiratory tract superinfections in the COVID-19 era: A retrospective quantitative analysis of antibiotic consumption and identification of antibiotic prescription drivers. *Intern. Emerg. Med.* **2022**, *17*, 141–151. [CrossRef]
8. Declercq, J.; A Van Damme, K.F.; De Leeuw, E.; Maes, B.; Bosteels, C.; Tavernier, S.J.; De Buyser, S.; Colman, R.; Hites, M.; Verschelden, G.; et al. Effect of anti-interleukin drugs in patients with COVID-19 and signs of cytokine release syndrome (COV-AID): A factorial, randomised, controlled trial. *Lancet Respir. Med.* **2021**, *9*, 1427–1438. [CrossRef]
9. Meschiari, M.; Onorato, L.; Bacca, E.; Orlando, G.; Menozzi, M.; Franceschini, E.; Bedini, A.; Cervo, A.; Santoro, A.; Sarti, M.; et al. Long-Term Impact of the COVID-19 Pandemic on In-Hospital Antibiotic Consumption and Antibiotic Resistance: A Time Series Analysis (2015–2021). *Antibiotics* **2022**, *11*, 826. [CrossRef]
10. Friedli, O.; Gasser, M.; Cusini, A.; Fulchini, R.; Vuichard-Gysin, D.; Tobler, R.H.; Wassilew, N.; Plüss-Suard, C.; Kronenberg, A. Impact of the COVID-19 Pandemic on Inpatient Antibiotic Consumption in Switzerland. *Antibiotics* **2022**, *11*, 792. [CrossRef]
11. Bartoletti, M.; Azap, O.; Barac, A.; Bussini, L.; Ergonul, O.; Krause, R.; Paño-Pardo, J.R.; Power, N.R.; Sibani, M.; Szabo, B.G.; et al. ESCMID COVID-19 living guidelines: Drug treatment and clinical management. *Clin. Microbiol. Infect.* **2022**, *28*, 222–238. [CrossRef]
12. World Health Organization (WHO). *Living Guidance for Clinical Management of COVID-19: Living Guidance*; World Health Organization (WHO): Geneva, Switzerland, 2021.
13. Alshaikh, F.S.; Godman, B.; Sindi, O.N.; Seaton, R.A.; Kurdi, A. Prevalence of bacterial coinfection and patterns of antibiotics prescribing in patients with COVID-19: A systematic review and meta-analysis. *PLoS ONE* **2022**, *17*, e0272375. [CrossRef]
14. Khan, S.; Bond, S.E.; Bakhit, M.; Hasan, S.S.; Sadeq, A.A.; Conway, B.R.; Aldeyab, M.A. COVID-19 Mixed Impact on Hospital Antimicrobial Stewardship Activities: A Qualitative Study in UK-Based Hospitals. *Antibiotics* **2022**, *11*, 1600. [CrossRef]
15. Fukushige, M.; Ngo, N.-H.; Lukmanto, D.; Fukuda, S.; Ohneda, O. Effect of the COVID-19 pandemic on antibiotic consumption: A systematic review comparing 2019 and 2020 data. *Front. Public Heal.* **2022**, *10*. [CrossRef]
16. Matteson, C.L.; Czaja, C.A.; Kronman, M.P.; Ziniel, S.; Parker, S.K.; Dodson, D.S. Impact of the coronavirus disease 2019 (COVID-19) pandemic on antimicrobial stewardship programs in Colorado hospitals. *Antimicrob Steward Healthc Epidemiol* **2022**, *2*, e172. [CrossRef]
17. Langford, B.J.; So, M.; Raybardhan, S.; Leung, V.; Westwood, D.; MacFadden, D.R.; Soucy, J.-P.R.; Daneman, N. Bacterial co-infection and secondary infection in patients with COVID-19: A living rapid review and meta-analysis. *Clin. Microbiol. Infect.* **2020**, *26*, 1622–1629. [CrossRef]
18. Lansbury, L.; Lim, B.; Baskaran, V.; Lim, W.S. Co-infections in people with COVID-19: A systematic review and meta-analysis. *J. Infect.* **2020**, *81*, 266–275. [CrossRef]
19. Russell, C.D.; Fairfield, C.J.; Drake, T.M.; Seaton, R.A.; Wootton, D.G.; Sigfrid, L.; Harrison, E.M.; Docherty, A.B.; I de Silva, T.; Egan, C.; et al. Co-infections, secondary infections, and antimicrobial use in patients hospitalised with COVID-19 during the first pandemic wave from the ISARIC WHO CCP-UK study: A multicentre, prospective cohort study. *Lancet Microbe* **2021**, *2*, e354–e365. [CrossRef]
20. Liew, Y.; Lee, W.; Tan, L.; Kwa, A.; Thien, S.; Cherng, B.; Chung, S.J. Antimicrobial stewardship programme: A vital resource for hospitals during the global outbreak of coronavirus disease 2019 (COVID-19). *Int. J. Antimicrob. Agents* **2020**, *56*, 106145. [CrossRef]
21. Huttner, B.; Catho, G.; Pao-Pardo, J.; Pulcini, C.; Schouten, J. COVID-19: Don't neglect antimicrobial stewardship principles! *Clin. Microbiol. Infect.* **2020**, *26*, 808–810. [CrossRef]
22. Staub, M.B.; Beaulieu, R.M.; Graves, J.; Nelson, G.E. Changes in antimicrobial utilization during the coronavirus disease 2019 (COVID-19) pandemic after implementation of a multispecialty clinical guidance team. *Infect. Control. Hosp. Epidemiol.* **2021**, *42*, 266–275. [CrossRef]
23. Venturini, S.; Avolio, M.; Fossati, S.; Callegari, A.; De Rosa, R.; Basso, B.; Zanusso, C.; Orso, D.; Cugini, F.; Crapis, M. Antimicrobial Stewardship in the Covid-19 Pandemic. *Hosp. Pharm.* **2022**, *57*, 416–418. [CrossRef]
24. Carrara, E.; Sibani, M.; Barbato, L.; Mazzaferri, F.; Salerno, N.D.; Conti, M.; Azzini, A.M.; Dalbeni, A.; Pellizzari, L.; Fontana, G.; et al. How to 'SAVE' antibiotics: Effectiveness and sustainability of a new model of antibiotic stewardship intervention in the internal medicine area. *Int J Antimicrob Agents.* **2022**, *60*, 106672. [CrossRef]

25. *The WHO AWaRe (Access, Watch, Reserve) Antibiotic Book*; World Health Organization: Geneva, Switzerland, 2022; Licence: CC BY-NC-SA 3.0 IGO.
26. Ponce-Alonso, M.; de la Fuente, J.S.; Rincón-Carlavilla, A.; Moreno-Nunez, P.; Martínez-García, L.; Escudero-Sánchez, R.; Pintor, R.; García-Fernández, S.; Cobo, J. Impact of the coronavirus disease 2019 (COVID-19) pandemic on nosocomial *Clostridioides difficile* infection. *Infect. Control. Hosp. Epidemiol.* **2021**, *42*, 406–410. [CrossRef]
27. Alberici, F.; Affatato, S.; Moratto, D.; Mescia, F.; Delbarba, E.; Guerini, A.; Tedesco, M.; Burbelo, P.; Zani, R.; Castagna, I.; et al. SARS-CoV-2 infection in dialysis and kidney transplant patients: Immunological and serological response. *J. Nephrol.* **2022**, *35*, 745–759. [CrossRef]
28. Guisado-Gil, A.B.; Infante-Domínguez, C.; Peñalva, G.; Praena, J.; Roca, C.; Navarro-Amuedo, M.D.; Aguilar-Guisado, M.; Espinosa-Aguilera, N.; Poyato-Borrego, M.; Romero-Rodríguez, N.; et al. Impact of the COVID-19 Pandemic on Antimicrobial Consumption and Hospital-Acquired Can-didemia and Multidrug-Resistant Bloodstream Infections. *Antibiotics* **2020**, *9*, 816. [CrossRef]
29. Pettit, N.; Nguyen, C.T.; Lew, A.; Bhagat, P.H.; Nelson, A.; Olson, G.; Ridgway, J.; Pho, M.; Pagkas-Bather, J. Reducing the use of empiric antibiotic therapy in COVID-19 on hospital admission. *BMC Infect. Dis.* **2021**, *21*, 516. [CrossRef]
30. Cong, W.; Stuart, B.; AIhusein, N.; Liu, B.; Tang, Y.-S.; Wang, H.; Wang, Y.; Manchundiya, A.; Lambert, H. Antibiotic Use and Bacterial Infection in COVID-19 Patients in the Second Phase of the SARS-CoV-2 Pandemic: A Scoping Review. *Antibiotics* **2022**, *11*, 991. [CrossRef]
31. Cecconi, M.; Piovani, D.; Brunetta, E.; Aghemo, A.; Greco, M.; Ciccarelli, M.; Angelini, C.; Voza, A.; Omodei, P.; Vespa, E.; et al. Early Predictors of Clinical Deterioration in a Cohort of 239 Patients Hospitalized for Covid-19 Infection in Lombardy, Italy. *J. Clin. Med.* **2020**, *9*, 1548. [CrossRef]
32. RECOVERY Collaborative Group (2021). Tocilizumab in patients admitted to hospital with COVID-19 (RECOVERY): A randomised, controlled, open-label, platform trial. *Lancet (London, England)* **2021**, *397*, 1637–1645. [CrossRef]
33. Masetti, C.; Generali, E.; Colapietro, F.; Voza, A.; Cecconi, M.; Messina, A.; Omodei, P.; Angelini, C.; Ciccarelli, M.; Badalamenti, S.; et al. High mortality in COVID-19 patients with mild respiratory disease. *Eur. J. Clin. Investig.* **2020**, *50*, e13314. [CrossRef] [PubMed]
34. Hasan, M.N.; Haider, N.; Stigler, F.L.; Khan, R.A.; McCoy, D.; Zumla, A.; Kock, R.A.; Uddin, J. The Global Case-Fatality Rate of COVID-19 Has Been Declining Since May 2020. *Am. J. Trop. Med. Hyg.* **2021**, *104*, 2176–2184. [CrossRef]
35. De Kraker, M.; Abbas, M.; Huttner, B.; Harbarth, S. Good epidemiological practice: A narrative review of appropriate scientific methods to evaluate the impact of antimicrobial stewardship interventions. *Clin. Microbiol. Infect.* **2017**, *23*, 819–825. [CrossRef] [PubMed]
36. WHO Collaborating Centre for Drug Statistics Methodology. *ATC Classification Index with DDDs, 2023*; WHO Collaborating Centre for Drug Statistics Methodology: Oslo, Norway, 2022.
37. Benić, M.S.; Milanič, R.; A Monnier, A.; Gyssens, I.C.; Adriaenssens, N.; Versporten, A.; Zanichelli, V.; Le Maréchal, M.; Huttner, B.; Tebano, G.; et al. Metrics for quantifying antibiotic use in the hospital setting: Results from a systematic review and international multidisciplinary consensus procedure. *J. Antimicrob. Chemother.* **2018**, *73*, vi50–vi58. [CrossRef] [PubMed]

Disclaimer/Publisher's Note: The statements, opinions and data contained in all publications are solely those of the individual author(s) and contributor(s) and not of MDPI and/or the editor(s). MDPI and/or the editor(s) disclaim responsibility for any injury to people or property resulting from any ideas, methods, instructions or products referred to in the content.

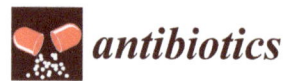

Article

Antibiotic Misuse Behaviours of Older People: Confirmation of the Factor Structure of the Antibiotic Use Questionnaire

Loni Schramm, Mitchell K. Byrne * and Taylor Sweetnam

Faculty of Health, Charles Darwin University, Darwin, NT 0909, Australia
* Correspondence: mitchell.byrne@cdu.edu.au

Abstract: Antibacterial resistance (AR) is responsible for steadily rising numbers of untreatable bacterial infections, most prevalently found in the older adult (OA) population due to age-related physical and cognitive deterioration, more frequent and long-lasting hospital visits, and reduced immunity. There are currently no established measures of antibiotic use behaviours for older adults, and theory-informed approaches to identifying the drivers of antibiotic use in older adults are lacking in the literature. The objective of this study was to identify predictors of antibiotic use and misuse in older adults using the Antibiotic Use Questionnaire (AUQ), a measure informed by the factors of the Theory of Planned Behaviour (TPB): attitudes and beliefs, social norms, perceived behavioural control, behaviour, and a covariate—knowledge. A measure of social desirability was included, and participants scoring highly were excluded to control for social desirability bias. Confirmatory Factor Analyses and regression analyses were conducted to test the hypotheses in a cross-sectional, anonymous survey. A total of 211 participants completed the survey, 47 of which were excluded due to incompletion and high social desirability scores (≥ 5). Results of the factor analysis confirmed that some (but not all) factors from previous research in the general population were confirmed in the OA sample. No factors were found to be significant predictors of antibiotic use behaviour. Several suggestions for the variance in results from that of the first study are suggested, including challenges with meeting requirement for statistical power. The paper concludes that further research is required to determine the validity of the AUQ in an older adult population.

Keywords: antibiotic misuse; older adults; Theory of Planned Behaviour; antimicrobial resistance; antibiotic stewardship

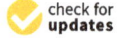

Citation: Schramm, L.; Byrne, M.K.; Sweetnam, T. Antibiotic Misuse Behaviours of Older People: Confirmation of the Factor Structure of the Antibiotic Use Questionnaire. *Antibiotics* **2023**, *12*, 718. https://doi.org/10.3390/antibiotics12040718

Academic Editors: Gyöngyvér Soós, Ria Benkő and Masafumi Seki

Received: 20 December 2022
Revised: 22 March 2023
Accepted: 28 March 2023
Published: 6 April 2023

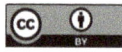

Copyright: © 2023 by the authors. Licensee MDPI, Basel, Switzerland. This article is an open access article distributed under the terms and conditions of the Creative Commons Attribution (CC BY) license (https://creativecommons.org/licenses/by/4.0/).

1. Introduction

1.1. Driving Factors of Antibiotic Resistance

Antimicrobial resistance (AMR), and in particular, antibiotic resistance (AR), is a growing concern in the health service provision [1]. AMR is described as the gradual changing of organisms—such as bacteria, viruses, fungi, and parasites—such that they become resistant to medicines and make infections harder to treat. These resistant organisms contribute to the spread of disease and chronic illness, and increase the risk of death [2]. There are heightened concerns around AR due to the apparent overuse of antibiotics in agricultural and medical settings [3]. The indiscriminate use of antibiotics is thought to be a driver of AR as bacterium develop defenses against antibiotics, resulting in a loss of efficiency in disease treatment [4].

AR contributes to increased mortality globally and is estimated to result in approximately 1600 Australian deaths annually [5]. As antibiotics become less effective, more infections will require the use of increasingly limited medical treatments or simply be untreatable [2]. The risk of AR infections and AR-related deaths is disproportionately higher for older adults due to their increased susceptibility to age-related comorbidities, making this population a high priority when conducting research on antibiotic use behaviours [6,7].

Currently, Australia's National Antimicrobial Resistance Strategy (NARS) has implemented multiple interventions into Australian healthcare systems in an attempt to reduce rates of unnecessary antibiotic use and increasing medical literacy amongst pharmacists and GPs [5,8]. Still, antibiotic use in Australia ranks highly amongst other wealthy countries, with prescribing rates in children approximately 30% higher than in the USA, and twice as high in adults (per capita) than Sweden [9,10]. Antibiotics are still frequently prescribed inappropriately for reasons unaligned with clinical practice guidelines. For example, 81% of Australian patients in 2017 received antibiotic prescriptions for upper respiratory tract infections, for which antibiotics are not recommended [1,11]. While prescriptions for antibiotics are decreasing annually, in 2019 over 26 million prescriptions were dispensed by GPs to at least 40.3% Australians [1]. Drivers of antibiotic misuse within the community include a lack of public health literacy and knowledge of AR/AMR, accessibility to non-prescribed antibiotics, and the level of stewardship involving healthcare professionals [4].

1.2. Public Health Literacy of AR and Prevalence of Antibiotic Use in Older Adults

Health literacy describes the skills and knowledge of a person regarding their health and healthcare systems [12]. It includes their ability to locate, interpret, and communicate health-related information, and use their knowledge of health services to seek appropriate care [12]. Lack of knowledge and awareness is a large contributor to the misuse of antibiotics and is predominantly determined by both education level and accessibility to public information [10]. In Machowski and Stålsby-Lundberg's (2019) review, 57% of Europeans in the general population were unaware of antibiotic ineffectiveness against viruses, 44% were unaware of ineffectiveness against colds and influenza, and approximately 20% considered it unlikely that AR would affect them or their family. The most common misconception regarding AR among older adults was that only humans (and not bacteria) become resistant to antibiotics with prolonged use, and therefore they would not contribute to AR [10]. Overall, older adults were more likely to overestimate their AR knowledge, with the belief that having previously taken specific antibiotics for familiar symptoms meant they could take them again—with or without a prescription [13,14]. Demographic predictors for antibiotic use behaviour varied by country: for some, use was reported as 7% higher for those less educated and 13% higher for those in worse economic circumstances, while other countries showed the opposite, with higher antibiotic use in higher-income families [15]. These findings suggest that population-specific health education strategies are essential for AR-focused interventions [7].

Older adults' health anxiety and health needs surpass those of younger people, and the incidence of GPs wrongly prescribing antibiotics is more frequent for older adults [16,17]. It is therefore particularly important to measure levels of health literacy and its influence on antibiotic use behaviours in this population [6]. Common health conditions frequently misconceived by older adults as requiring a prescription for antibiotics include upper respiratory tract infections, urinary tract infections, seeking relief from pain symptoms, and common colds and flu [18–20]. These misconceptions are likely driven from fear of an increased risk to health, and worsening age-related health issues [21]. Compared to younger adult age groups, clinical presentations of atypical infections, rapid disease progression, risk of inappropriate treatment, and prolonged recovery periods are more common in older adults, whose risk of exposure to AR is heightened if they live alone with limited access to health information [22,23].

1.3. Antibiotic Misuse and Stewardship in Older Adults

According to the World Health Organization (WHO) (2021), inappropriate use of antibiotics occurs when they are obtained or prescribed without appropriate diagnosis as treatment for symptoms not included in the health guidelines, in doses that are excessive (i.e., with treatment courses longer than the infection requires), with unnecessary repeat prescriptions, and/or when antibiotic treatment information and risks are not adequately communicated to the patient. Non-prescription antibiotic use, non-adherence to antibiotic use guidelines, and antibiotic hoarding are classified as misuse of antibiotics [24]. Despite the WHO declaring antibiotics a prescription-only medicine and limiting their use to specific conditions, research indicates that sociocultural, behavioural, and economic factors influence antibiotic use that violates recommended guidelines [1,3]. Four major factors relating to the misuse of antibiotics commonly identified globally in the literature include: lack of health literacy regarding AR; ease of access to antibiotics without a prescription; the role of health practitioners in providing prescriptions; and incomplete treatment courses leading to the accumulation of leftover antibiotics [25].

Consumption of leftover antibiotics from earlier prescriptions is one of many antibiotic misuse behaviours that are more likely to occur in older adults who may have limited resources and inadequate health literacy regarding appropriate antibiotic use [20]. Reasons for antibiotic misuse amongst older adults included having more medication than needed, feeling better, experiencing side effects, forgetting to take them, or feeling no difference in symptoms, with over 65% of older adults keeping their leftover antibiotics for themselves [20]. Additional research in the US, UK, Asia, and Africa suggests that over one-third of antibiotic treatment courses/regimens are not adhered to in the general population—50% prematurely cease adherence to antibiotic treatment when improved, and one-third store leftover antibiotics for themselves or others' future use [26,27].

The use of non-prescription antibiotics has also been influenced by an increased use of technology, with evidence showing that telehealth sessions with a GP are associated with a diminished capability to accurately diagnose and provide appropriate advice about the use of antibiotics [28,29]. The availability of antibiotics being obtained through unauthorized websites, or social media platforms, is also related to technological advances [30]. An Australian investigation of consumer demand for non-prescription medications by Hope et al. (2020) found that 71% of pharmacists were asked by customers for non-prescription access to antibiotics daily or weekly. Up to 75% of pharmacists considered down-scheduling antibiotics to non-prescription status, indicating that increased training in AR-related stewardship policies for pharmacists is required [31].

1.4. Theory of Planned Behaviour

Multiple studies have used the Theory of Planned Behaviour (TPB) to try and explain antibiotic use behaviours, with evidence suggesting that it can explain large proportions of previously unexplained variance in these behaviours [4,32]. The TPB suggests three components predict intention to act: perceived behavioural control (PBC), attitudes and beliefs, and subjective norms [33]. Thus, the TPB can be used to identify behavioural, motivational, and social factors that influence intention to misuse antibiotics (Figure 1) [4,34–36]. Indeed, Byrne et al. (2019) found that behavioural intention for antibiotic use could be predicted by the three TPB factors, and that knowledge of antibiotic use and AR significantly influenced attitudes and beliefs. The authors developed the Antibiotics Use Questionnaire (AUQ) in consultation with a multidisciplinary panel of experts from fields including psychology, business, and heath. Following the analysis of 293 responses, eighteen items of the questionnaire were retained that reflected the three variables of the TPB, the outcome variable of behaviour, and the covariate of knowledge. The results indicated that antibiotic use behaviour could be significantly explained by each of the variables, and that the TPB model explained 70% of the variance in antibiotic use and misuse.

1.5. Aim

The aim of the present study is to replicate the factor structure from Byrne et al. (2019) within an older adult population. Should the factor structure be confirmed, the study then seeks to investigate if the AUQ has the capacity to predict behavioural intentions of antibiotic use and misuse in older adults using TPB constructs. It is hypothesized that knowledge and intention to use antibiotics will be positively associated with the TPB factors, replicating the findings of previous research [4].

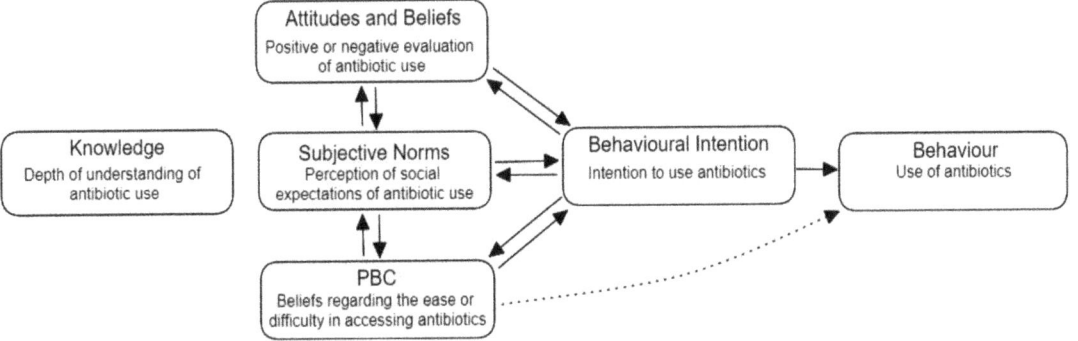

Figure 1. Theory of Planned Behaviour Model, adapted from Ajzen (1991) [35].

2. Materials and Methods

2.1. Participants and Procedure

To be eligible for the study, participants were required to live independently within their community, be over 70 years of age, and have no known history of cognitive deficits. The criteria of 70 years of age was selected over the usual older adult age-range of 65, as recent research suggests that due to medical and technological advancements in health, older adults are increasingly more independent, have less subjective cognitive decline, and are overall healthier at older ages [37–39]. A power analysis for confirmatory factor analysis (CFA) was conducted using the statistical programming language R [40]. The semPower package [41] was used for the calculation, with power set at 0.8, alpha at 0.05, an estimated degree of freedom of 148, and a root mean square error of approximation (RMSEA) of 0.5. This estimated that at least 132 participants were required for our CFA [41].

Recruitment was undertaken via purposive sampling to identify individuals meeting eligibility criteria. A total of 110 participants were recruited within the Darwin community (Northern Australia) and surveyed in-person by the first author (labelled the 'In-Person' group). Recruitment took place at local community venues, social events, and local independent living facilities for older adults. Ten participants in this group were given the survey in hard-copy and completed it without the researcher present, returning it via pre-paid mail. Participation was incentivized by entering all participant into a randomly drawn raffle for a $50 Woolworths gift voucher. Eight 'in-person' participants were excluded due to incompletion of the survey, leaving 102 persons in this sample. While most 'in-person' participants self-completed the survey, 26% of the 'in-person' group requested help (labelled as 'had-help') to complete it due to issues with reading ability and/or physical impairments such as arthritis. For this group, questions were read aloud to the participant and/or the survey was completed on behalf of the participant by the researcher as they provided their answers.

To increase the sample size in line with our power calculation, an additional 93 participants were recruited using the online crowdsourcing platform M-Turk (labelled 'M-Turk' group). This group completed the survey online via the survey platform Qualtrics, with an incentive of $2.00 in Amazon credit for completion of the survey. Bots were controlled for by a forced-response question requiring visual logic ability ('what is the third word in the following sentence?'). Both groups provided informed consent before participation. This study was conducted in accordance with the National Statement on Ethical Conduct in Human Research and approved by the Charles Darwin University Human Research Ethics Committee (approval no. H22041).

2.2. Measures

The Antibiotics Use Questionnaire (AUQ) [4] includes a total of 30 items measured using either dichotomous response options (true or false) or a 4-point Likert scale (strongly agree, agree, disagree, and strongly disagree). Six demographic items are included that measure age, gender (male, female, or other), education (primary school, did not complete secondary school, completed secondary school, TAFE, bachelor's degree, or Post-Graduate Degree), health training, having friends or family in health work, and postcode. Two items are included for subjective norms (i.e., 'my friends and family only use antibiotics when prescribed'); four items each are included for behavioural intention, knowledge, PBC, and attitudes and beliefs (i.e., 'it is my right to ask for antibiotics from my doctor'); and six items randomly selected from the Marlowe–Crowne Social Desirability Scale (SDS) are used to measure the honesty and reliability of answers [42]. The knowledge factor assesses the general understanding of antibiotic use and proximity or accessibility to sources of health information (e.g., 'antibiotics are needed for the common cold'). The AUQ does not directly measure antibiotic use or behaviour but does measure behavioural intentions related to antibiotic use and misuse (i.e., 'I would take antibiotics without consulting a doctor'). Please see the Supplementary Materials for a copy of the AUQ (Supplementary Material Measure S1).

2.3. Statistical Analysis

All analyses were performed using the statistical software jamovi (version 2.3.9.0) [42]. Initial descriptive analyses and an independent sample *t*-tests were used to compare the In-Person and M-Turk samples. Replicating the strategy used by Byrne et al. (2019), a CFA using orthogonal principal component analysis with varimax rotation was used to confirm the five-factor structure of the AUQ in our sample. Model fit was assessed with several fit metrics including the Comparative Fit Index (CFI), Tucker–Lewis Index (TLI), and RMSEA. CFI and TLI values above 0.95 and RMSEA values below 0.08 were used to indicate good fit to the data [43]. To identify predictors of antibiotic use, an ordinary least-squares regression analysis was used with the behaviour factor (i.e., intention to use antibiotics) of the AUQ as the outcome variable. The predictors included in the model were the three TPB factors (subjective norms, PBC, attitudes and beliefs), demographic variables, and social desirability scores. The knowledge factor was included as a covariate, to replicate prior research [5,34,37].

3. Results

3.1. Initial Findings

Descriptive analyses found that participants' mean age was 74.3 years ($SD = 3.98$) and their mean education level was a TAFE qualification ($SD = 1.40$). Social desirability scores showed that 19% ($N = 39$) of all respondents scored ≥ 5 points ($M = 3.75$, $SD = 1.03$), and these were subsequently excluded from the data, leaving 164 participants in total.

Upon closer analysis, the M-Turk and In-Person groups showed significant mean differences in the education level, age, health training, and health worker in the family factors (Table 1).

Using an Independent Samples T-Test, 14 TPB items out of the 18 also showed significant differences in overall mean scores, with a Mann–Whitney-U test significant in 12 out of 18 items and Shapiro Wilk significant for all items, suggesting a violation of normality (see Table 2).

Due to the significant differences between groups, the results of the CFA were conducted only on the In-Person group, the descriptive statistics of which are reported in Table 3.

The In-Person group included two subgroups: Had Help ($N = 21$), or Self-Completed ($N = 58$). Within the In-Person group, 10 TPB items showed differences in mean scores between subgroups for social desirability, with the subgroup that had help demonstrating a higher mean ($M = 3.14$, $SD = 0.806$) than the group that self-completed the survey ($M = 3.43$, $SD = 0.507$).

Table 1. Mean Differences Between Groups.

	Survey Platform	N	Mean	SD	T-Statistic	p-Value
Education	In-Person	79	3.49	1.395	−9.69	<0.001
	M-Turk	85	5.19	0.779		
Healthcare Training	In-Person	79	1.80	0.404	10.09	<0.001
	M-Turk	85	1.18	0.383		
Healthcare Worker in Family	In-Person	79	1.47	0.502	5.61	<0.001
	M-Turk	85	1.11	0.310		
Age	In-Person	79	76.65	4.139	8.90	<0.001
	M-Turk	85	72.09	2.175		

Table 2. Independent Samples T-Test—Mann–Whitney U For TPB Items.

		Statistic	p
Q1. Abs Reduce Cold Symptoms	Mann-Whitney U	3275	0.760
Q2. Friends & Family Follow AB Recommendations	Mann-Whitney U	824	<0.001
Q3. Abs Are Needed for Colds	Mann-Whitney U	3350	0.978
Q4. Abs Can Have Negative Side Effects	Mann-Whitney U	855	<0.001
Q5. I Use Abs Without Dr. Consultation	Mann-Whitney U	3162	0.490
Q6. I Use Leftover Abs	Mann-Whitney U	3217	0.619
Q7. It's My Right to Ask for ABs	Mann-Whitney U	819	<0.001
Q8. Friends & Family	Mann-Whitney U	1037	<0.001
Q.9 Know When I Need AB's	Mann-Whitney U	2158	<0.001
Q10. Use of ABs Without Prescription is Common	Mann-Whitney U	1952	<0.001
Q11. Confident to Ask for AB's	Mann-Whitney U	995	<0.001
Q12. Abs Will be Less Effective in Future	Mann-Whitney U	970	<0.001
Q13. I Consult Dr. Prior to Taking ABs	Mann-Whitney U	417	<0.001
Q14. I Keep Leftover ABs	Mann-Whitney U	2878	0.090
Q15. Easily Get Abs from Dr.	Mann-Whitney U	1465	<0.001
Q16. Easily Get Abs Online	Mann-Whitney U	2717	0.018
Q17. Easily Get Abs Family	Mann-Whitney U	3147	0.438
Q18. Expect Abs from Dr.	Mann-Whitney U	2553	0.004

Table 3. In-Person Group Descriptive Statistics for Demographics and TPB.

	Self-Completed or Had Help	Mean	SD
Gender	Self-Completed	1.67	0.482
	Had Help	1.57	0.535
Education	Self-Completed	3.71	1.654
	Had Help	2.57	0.976
Age	Self-Completed	78.17	3.435
	Had Help	80.43	5.593
Health Training	Self-Completed	1.83	0.387
	Had Help	1.86	0.378
Health Worker in Family	Self-Completed	1.50	0.511
	Had Help	1.71	0.488
Behaviour	Self-Completed	2.14	0.410
	Had Help	2.54	0.419
Social Desirability Scale	Self-Completed	5.13	0.338
	Had Help	5.00	0.000
Knowledge	Self-Completed	2.58	0.319
	Had Help	2.64	0.378
Attitudes and Beliefs	Self-Completed	2.54	0.588
	Had Help	2.79	0.585
Subjective Norms	Self-Completed	2.98	0.454
	Had Help	2.86	0.244
Perceived Behavioural Control	Self-Completed	1.82	0.486
	Had Help	2.04	0.304

3.2. CFA of the AUQ

Items loading significantly onto relative factors are displayed in Figure 2, showing item loading scores ranging between 0.39 and 0.88 ($p \leq 0.05$). The fit statistics indicated that the TPB model was a mediocre fit to the data ($\chi^2 = 231$, $p \leq 0.001$; CFI = 0.74; TLI = 0.68; RMSEA = 0.10). While the factor structure was confirmed, not all items fit well onto the factor structure, with multiple response items loading significantly onto several factors. Table 4 highlights in red any standardized estimates above 3 to identify items that fit into multiple factors.

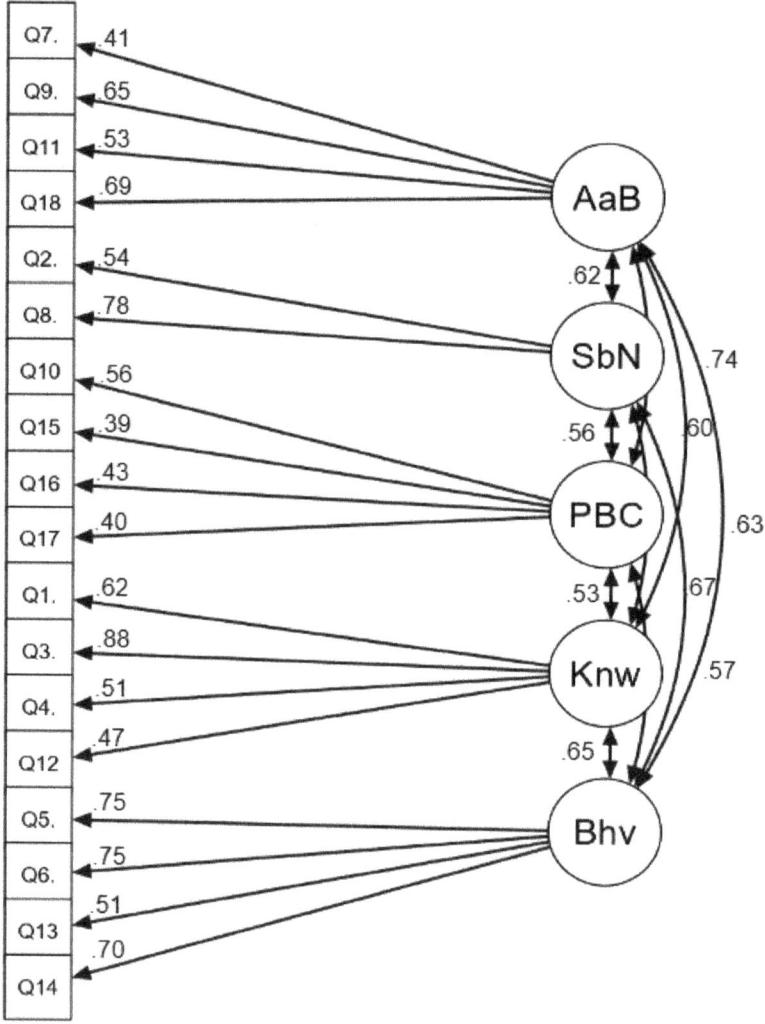

Figure 2. Results of CFA on AUQ factors with standardized parameter estimates. Key: AaB = Attitudes and Beliefs, SbN = Subjective Norms, Knw = Knowledge, Bhv = Behaviour.

Despite exclusion of the three items that loaded significantly on three or more factors, the fit of the factor loadings remained mediocre. Cronbach's Alpha demonstrated modest but acceptable internal reliability for both groups (M-Turk and In-Person) for all factors (Table 5).

Table 4. CFA Modification Indices for In-Person Group Factor Loadings.

	Attitudes & Beliefs	Subjective Norms	Perceived Behavioural Control	Knowledge	Behaviour
Q7. It's My Right to Ask for ABs		0.508	0.227	2.207	0.048
Q9. Know When I Need ABs		1.209	3.894	0.301	1.371
Q11. Confident to Ask for ABs		5.325	7.097	0.817	4.715
Q18. Expect Abs form Dr.		5.955	20.565	5.336	10.053
Q2. Friends & Family Follow AB Recommendations	4.164		1.178	1.368	3.140
Q8. Friends & Family Only Use Prescribed ABs	4.164		1.178	1.368	3.140
Q10. Use of Abs Without Prescription is Common	0.798	3.309		1.885	3.664
Q15. Easily Get Abs from Dr.	6.717	0.014		0.001	9.237
Q16. Easily Get Abs Online	10.109	5.341		5.631	3.962
Q17. Easily Get Abs Family	0.087	3.224		0.581	7.848
Q1. Abs Reduce Cold Symptoms	0.002	2.682	0.664		2.476
Q3. Abs Are Needed for Colds	0.907	0.174	0.180		0.375
Q4. Abs Can Have Negative Side Effects	3.221	0.007	0.002		0.025
Q12. Abs Will be Less Effective in Future	0.235	2.674	3.329		7.758
Q5. I Use Abs Without Dr. Consultation	0.018	0.006	1.675	5.455	
Q6. I Use Leftover ABs	1.386	0.452	0.064	1.434	
Q13. I Consult Dr. Prior to Taking ABs	0.059	0.233	0.609	0.048	
Q14. I Keep Leftover ABs	1.693	0.109	1.179	1.893	

Table 5. Reliability and Descriptive Statistics for TPB Scales.

	Survey Platform	Mean	SD	Cronbach's α
Behaviour	In-Person	2.76	0.56	0.68
	M-Turk	2.32	0.69	0.77
Knowledge	In-Person	3.03	0.53	0.70
	M-Turk	2.73	0.54	0.53
Perceived Behavioural Control	In-Person	2.02	0.40	0.48
	M-Turk	2.03	0.53	0.59
Subjective Norms	In-Person	2.83	0.55	0.59
	M-Turk	2.86	0.76	0.75
Attitudes & Beliefs	In-Person	2.76	0.56	0.68
	M-Turk	2.32	0.69	0.77

3.3. Regression Analyses for the SDS, AUQ Factors and Behaviour

A regression analysis was completed using item means of the outcome variable Behaviour and the AUQ factors within the In-Person group, which found that none of the TPB factors significantly predicted behavioural intention (adjusted $R^2 \leq 0.3, p \geq 0.05$). This was the same for items measuring social desirability (adjusted $R^2 = 0.20, p \geq 0.001$). Individually, the item related to healthcare training ($\beta = 0.42, p \leq 0.001$), the two PBC items (Q.10 and Q.17), two knowledge items (Q.3 and Q.12), and one attitude and belief item (Q.1) were found to interact with the outcome variable related to behavioural intentions ($\beta = 0.25$–$0.40, p \leq 0.05$). The Shapiro–Wilks test was significant ($p \leq 0.71$), and VIF indicated low collinearity (VIF ≤ 1.7).

4. Discussion

4.1. Predictors of Antibiotic Misuse Behaviours

The present study aimed to replicate the factor structure of the Antibiotics Use Questionnaire designed by Byrne et al. [4] in a local, community-based Northern Territorian older adult population. The study additionally aimed to investigate if the AUQ has the capacity to predict behavioural intentions of antibiotic use and misuse in older adults using TPB constructs, with the inclusion of knowledge of AMR as a covariate.

The required sample size proved difficult to obtain, leading to the recruitment of additional OA participants via M-Turk to meet the sample size requirements for a CFA. This resulted in data from a second OA group being analyzed, whose mean demographic and social desirability scores differed significantly from those of the local community-based older adults. As the present study's aim was to obtain a cohort of verifiably independently living and local older adults whose age and cognitive function was verified through face-to-face administration of the AUQ in public community venues, the M-Turk group was selected for exclusion (in comparison) due to greater relevance of the In-Person group's demographics to the study's inclusion criteria.

4.2. Comparison with Previous Research

The TPB factor structure from the original study by Byrne et al. (2019) was confirmed in the current study's local OA population; however, the poor fit of some items to the factor structure indicates that the structure and items of the AUQ may require adaptation to ensure its generalizability to an OA population. This is supported by comparing the 43% of participants in the Byrne et al. [4] study being less than 24 years of age and 58% having reported as having a bachelor's degree or higher, indicating a significant difference in demographics between the original and current studies' target populations. These cohort variances may explain differences in item loadings. An alternative explanation of the variance in results may be that the current study's sample size was limited to 60% of the required number of participants for the CFA. When compared between studies, items that loaded poorly within the factor structure in the current study also showed small factor loadings in the previous study (with standardized estimate coefficients between 0.41 and 0.52), suggesting further research is needed to establish more consistent results using the AUQ [4].

Findings from the regression analysis, hypothesized to replicate Byrne et al.'s (2019) research, found no association between the factors of the TPB, knowledge, or social desirability items and behavioural intentions of antibiotic use, suggesting that in an OA population, the AUQ is unable to reliably predict behavioural intention using factors of the TPB. This contradicts the previous study's findings, which found that TPB constructs explained 70% of the variance in behavioural intentions related to antibiotic use [5]. Comparatively, Byrne et al. [4] found that demographic variables did not significantly predict behavioural intention in their sample, whereas healthcare training showed a significant interaction with behavioural intention in the current study—although similar in both studies, no other demographic variable was significantly correlated with behavioural intention. The lack of correlation between the TPB factors of the AUQ and antibiotic use behaviour in the current study may again be explained by the small sample size, or the differences in population demographics between the two studies that potentially render the current version of the AUQ unsuitable for use with older adults [4]. Contradictory to the current study and the study conducted by Byrne et al. [4], other research has found significant predictors of antibiotic use in demographic variables. For example, research has found that having a healthcare worker as a friend or family member was associated with increased antibiotic misuse [44–46]. These discrepancies in the findings further suggest the potential generalizability and/or effect size issues with the population sample of the current and the previous replicated study [4].

4.3. Older Adults and TPB Factors

Factors of the TPB model must be recognised as defining different areas of behavioural intention for older adults, whose social, emotional, and economical contexts can differ substantially from the younger populations [38]. In particular, PBC for older adults constitutes a different factor within the TPB than for the younger population: physiological impairment is a significant barrier to PBC and health-related self-efficacy, as conditions such as dementia, arthritis, heart disease, hearing loss, and diabetes largely affect mental health, mobility, diet and nutrition, memory, and sleep [47–49]. These issues can impact the independence of older adults, preventing them from driving, self-care, and essential self-maintenance behaviours such as regular medication adherence [50]. Psychological issues such as depression, anxiety, and prolonged grief are also common in older adults due to these limiting and significant physiological, social, and environmental changes in themselves and their relationships with loved ones [51]. Additionally, ageism reported in research experienced by older adults in GP clinics and other healthcare settings, such as pharmacies and hospitals, is suggested to affect the self-efficacy of older adults in being able to communicate their needs effectively, and to feel supported and informed by healthcare professionals [52]. PBC in accessing and using antibiotics with or without a prescription, and adherence to appropriate guidelines for antibiotics, are likely to be impacted by each of these factors for older adults, and in turn, affect attitudes and beliefs about their antibiotic use, as well as subjective norms when relating to others.

The concept that PBC has greater influence on behavioural intention for older adults contradicts previous research utilizing the TPB, which typically weights the TPB constructs equally. However, it has been suggested that there is potential that PBC may serve as a moderating variable for attitudes and beliefs and subjective norms [34,37,53]. A study by La Barbera and colleagues [36] found that levels of PBC were positively associated with attitudes and beliefs, and both negatively and positively associated with subjective norms. This suggestion may explain the results in the original study by Byrne et al. [4], which found that subjective norms had the weakest internal consistency compared to other factors and contained only two items. This is supported by findings from Castanier et al. (2013), who found that higher PBC was correlated with lower subjective norms (i.e., people who felt more in control were less likely to be influenced by peer pressure) [54]. These findings may relate to the current sample of older adults, in that the participants selected were assumed to have higher-than-average PBC for their age group due to their active, engaged, and independent participation in social clubs and events. Additionally, Sussman and Gifford (2019) suggest the TPB can be interpreted as having a reverse-causal relationship, with behaviour being influenced by the three base factors [53]. These potentially multidirectional interactions between behavioural intention, knowledge, and PBC for older adults and health beliefs may provide an additional alternative explanation for the differences in factor structure loadings between the current study and the previous study by Byrne et al. (2019) [4]. More broadly speaking, it may also provide further evidence of the complexities of older adults' choices and experiences regarding antibiotic use behaviours that must be considered when constructing or adapting health behaviour intervention measures and strategies for this population.

4.4. Strengths and Limitations

The current study benefited from the inclusion of a widely representative sample of OA participants from all areas within the local community and from a wide range of cultural backgrounds represented in Australia's Northern Territory. Limitations of this study include the challenges with obtaining an adequate sample size due to the low numbers of independent and accessible local Northern-Territorian older adults. Furthermore, the differences between the data collected through M-Turk and in person resulted in the exclusion of participants recruited online, resulting in a smaller sample size being used than what was required for a CFA.

Similarly, there was a potential for bias due to differences in cognitive ability, as the current study did not include controls for diagnosed cognitive deficits or decline. Differentiating these from naturally occurring, age-related subjective cognitive decline is recognised as a complex issue in self-reported health behaviour research involving older adults [55,56]; however, the inclusion of appropriate measures was beyond the scope of the current study. Issues with validity related to the social desirability also arose, given that the measure was self-reported, leading to a higher likelihood of falsified responses [57] within the In-Person group. The subgroup that was assisted with their survey responses demonstrated higher scores for social desirability bias than the group that completed the survey themselves, indicating that the assistance of the researcher likely resulted in increased social desirability. Therefore, despite the benefit of increased survey accessibility due to researcher assistance in completion of the survey, this assistance may have skewed the data.

Lastly, the differences in perceived behavioural control compared to actual behavioural control limits the ability to predict antibiotic use behaviour from intentions. It should also be noted that intention to act on a behaviour does not guarantee the behaviour will be acted upon (for example, people are unlikely to use antibiotics unless they are sick enough or feel they need them, regardless of their intentions).

5. Conclusions

The primary aim of the study was to replicate the factor structure from Byrne et al. (2019) [4] within an older adult population. Results from the current study show that this factor structure is indeed confirmed. Despite these results, limitations due to sample size and accessibility restricted the generalizability and validity of results, and no correlation was found between behavioural intention and antibiotic use behaviours. Further research is required to adapt AUQ items specifically for older adults and confirm this factor structure in OA populations with a larger sample size, in-person recruitment, and more accessible and efficient AUQ delivery. More accessible methods of conducting the survey are recommended for this age group, such as assisted electronic delivery via tablet, where questions are pre-recorded to be played out loud if needed, which would control for social desirability bias found in the current study. Additionally, accounting for the differences in PBC in the OA population is suggested when adapting items to better measure antibiotic use behaviours in older adults. Finally, future research involving older adults would benefit from measures controlling for cognitive decline, such as a test of grip strength, which has been shown to have good predictive validity, and the addition to the AUQ of an item requesting an indication of severity of self-identified subjective cognitive decline [58]. Overall, these results suggest that the AUQ has the potential to become a valuable tool to measure behavioural intentions for antibiotic use in older adults and supports research that suggests that age-specific training and transparency regarding information on AMR is required by health service providers when treating older adults.

Supplementary Materials: The following supporting information can be downloaded at: https://www.mdpi.com/article/10.3390/antibiotics12040718/s1. Measure S1: The Antibiotic Use Questionnaire.

Author Contributions: L.S.: Conceptualization, data curation, formal analysis, funding acquisition, investigation, methodology, project administration, writing—original draft, and writing—review & editing. M.K.B.: Conceptualization, funding acquisition, supervision, and writing—review & editing. T.S.: writing—review and editing. All authors have read and agreed to the published version of the manuscript.

Funding: There was no external funding associated with this research.

Institutional Review Board Statement: This study was conducted in accordance with the National Statement on Ethical Conduct in Human Research, and approved by the CDU Human Research Ethics Committee, ethics committee of Charles Darwin University, Australia (ethics code H22041, granted on 6 June 2022).

Informed Consent Statement: Informed consent was obtained from all subjects involved in the study.

Data Availability Statement: The data presented in this study are available on request from the corresponding author. The data are not publicly available due to the potential for participant identification.

Acknowledgments: Thank you to the following events, venues and services that permitted face-to-face recruitment for 118 local participants in the Northern Territory: The Palmerston Over 50 Club, the Palmerston Recreation Centre, Pearl Aged Care Independent Living, the Darwin Senior Citizens

Club, the Darwin Senior's Expo, COTA NT, Darwin Bowls Club, PROBUS Casuarina, the Darwin Chung Wah Society, the Pensioner's Workshop Association, the Alice Springs Seniors Coordinating Committee, Alice Springs Bridge Club, and Flynn Lodge Independent Living; and to Pam McLennan for contributions of invaluable administrative and technical support. CRediT statement above made using the online tool Tenzing by Holcombe et al., 2020 [59].

Conflicts of Interest: The authors declare no conflict of interest.

References

1. Australian Commission on Safety and Quality in Health Care. *Aura: Fourth Australian Report on Antimicrobial Use and Resistance in Human Health*; Australian Government: Sydney, NSW, Australia, 2021.
2. World Health Organisation. *Antimocrobial Resistance Fact Sheet*; World Health Organisation: Geneva, Switzerland, 2021.
3. World Health Organisation. *Tracss Country Report on the Implementation of National Action Plan on Antimicrobial Resistance (AMR): Australia*; World Health Organisation: Geneva, Switzerland, 2021.
4. Byrne, M.K.; Miellet, S.; McGlinn, A.; Fish, J.; Meedya, S.; Reynolds, N.; van Oijen, A.M. The drivers of antibiotic use and misuse: The development and investigation of a theory driven community measure. *BMC Public Health* **2019**, *19*, 1425. [CrossRef]
5. Van-Driel, M.; Gregory, M.; Emma, B.; Jonathan, D.; Lisa, H.; Clare, H. Preserving antibiotics for the future. *Aust. J. Gen. Pract.* **2022**, *51*, 10–13. [CrossRef] [PubMed]
6. Kong, L.S.; Islahudin, F.; Muthupalaniappen, L.; Chong, W.W. Knowledge and expectations on antibiotic use among older adults in Malaysia: A cross-sectional survey. *Geriatrics* **2019**, *4*, 61. [CrossRef] [PubMed]
7. Guo, H.; Hildon, Z.J.-L.; Lye, D.C.B.; Straughan, P.T.; Chow, A. The associations between poor antibiotic and antimicrobial resistance knowledge and inappropriate antibiotic use in the general population are modified by age. *Antibiotics* **2022**, *11*, 47. [CrossRef] [PubMed]
8. Department of Health and Agriculture. Australia's national antimicrobial resistance strategy—2020 and beyond. In *Agriculture DoHa*; Commonwealth of Australia: Canberra, ACT, Australia, 2019.
9. Anderson, R.; Rhodes, A.; Cranswick, N.; Downes, M.; O'Hara, J.; Measey, M.-A.; Gwee, A. A nationwide parent survey of antibiotic use in Australian children. *J. Antimicrob. Chemother.* **2020**, *75*, 1347–1351. [CrossRef]
10. Hawkins, O.; Scott, A.M.; Montgomery, A.; Nicholas, B.; Mullan, J.; van Oijen, A.; Degeling, C. Comparing public attitudes, knowledge, beliefs and behaviours towards antibiotics and antimicrobial resistance in Australia, United Kingdom, and Sweden (2010-2021): A systematic review, meta-analysis, and comparative policy analysis. *PLoS ONE* **2022**, *17*, 110–123. [CrossRef]
11. World Health Organisation. *WHO Essential Medicines List Antibiotic Book—Infographics—Version 1.1*; World Health Organisation: Geneva, Switzerland, 2021; pp. 1–141.
12. Liu, C.; Wang, D.; Liu, C.; Jiang, J.; Wang, X.; Chen, H.; Ju, X.; Zhang, X. What is the meaning of health literacy? A systematic review and qualitative synthesis. *Fam. Med. Community Health* **2020**, *8*, 251–264. [CrossRef]
13. Grigoryan, L.; Germanos, G.; Zoorob, R.; Juneja, S.; Raphael, J.; Paasche-Orlow, M.; Trautner, B. Use of antibiotics without a prescription in the U.S. population. *Ann. Intern. Med.* **2019**, *171*, 257–263. [CrossRef]
14. Smith, C.A.; Chang, E.; Gallego, G.; Khan, A.; Armour, M.; Balneaves, L.G. An education intervention to improve decision making and health literacy among older Australians: A randomised controlled trial. *BMC Geriatr.* **2019**, *19*, 129–140. [CrossRef]
15. Machowska, A.; Stålsby-Lundborg, C. Drivers of Irrational Use of Antibiotics in Europe. *Int. J. Environ. Res. Public Health* **2019**, *16*, 27. [CrossRef]
16. Cattaneo, D.; Falcone, M.; Gervasoni, C.; Marriott, D.J.E. Therapeutic drug monitoring of antibiotics in the elderly: A narrative review. *Ther. Drug Monit.* **2022**, *44*, 75–85. [CrossRef]
17. Dylis, A.; Boureau, A.S.; Coutant, A.; Batard, E.; Javaudin, F.; Berrut, G.; de Decker, L.; Chapelet, G. Antibiotics prescription and guidelines adherence in elderly: Impact of the comorbidities. *BMC Geriatr.* **2019**, *19*, 291. [CrossRef]
18. Cox, S.; Lo-A-Foe, K.; van Hoof, M.; Dinant, G.-J.; Oudhuis, G.; Savelkoul, P.; Cals, J.; de Bont, E. Physician-targeted interventions in antibiotic prescribing for urinary tract infections in general practice: A systematic review. *Antibiotics* **2022**, *11*, 1560. [CrossRef]
19. Gajdács, M.; Ábrók, M.; Lázár, A.; Burián, K. Urinary tract infections in elderly patients: A 10-year study on their epidemiology and antibiotic resistance based on the WHO Access, Watch and Reserve (AWaRe) classification. *Antibiotics* **2021**, *10*, 1098. [CrossRef] [PubMed]
20. Malani, P.; Solway, E.; Kirch, M.; Singer, D.C.; Kullgren, J.T. Use and perceptions of antibiotics among US adults aged 50–80 years. *Infect. Control Hosp. Epidemiol.* **2021**, *42*, 628–629. [CrossRef] [PubMed]
21. Manafo, E.; Wong, S. Health literacy programs for older adults: A systematic literature review. *Health Educ. Res.* **2012**, *27*, 947–960. [CrossRef] [PubMed]
22. Beckett, C.L.; Harbarth, S.; Huttner, B. Special considerations of antibiotic prescription in the geriatric population. *Clin. Microbiol. Infect.* **2015**, *21*, 3–9. [CrossRef]
23. Raban, M.Z.; Gates, P.J.; Gasparini, C.; Westbrook, J.I. Temporal and regional trends of antibiotic use in long-term aged care facilities across 39 countries, 1985-2019: Systematic review and meta-analysis. *PLoS ONE* **2021**, *16*, 225–234. [CrossRef]
24. O'Neill, J. *Tackling Drug-Resistant Infections Globally: Final Report and Recommendations*; Government of the United Kingdom: London, UK, 2016.

25. Merlino, J.; Siarakas, S. Antibiotic prescribing and antimicrobial resistance from an Australian perspective. *Microb. Drug Resist.* **2022**, *1*, 10–22. [CrossRef]
26. Morgan, D.J.; Okeke, I.N.; Laxminarayan, R.; Perencevich, E.N.; Weisenberg, S. Non-prescription antimicrobial use worldwide: A systematic review. *Lancet Infect. Dis.* **2011**, *11*, 692–701. [CrossRef]
27. Sun, R.; Yao, T.; Zhou, X.; Harbarth, S.; Lin, L. Non-biomedical factors affecting antibiotic use in the community: A mixed-methods systematic review and meta-analysis. *Clin. Microbiol. Infect.* **2022**, *28*, 345–354. [CrossRef] [PubMed]
28. Peters, L.; Greenfield, G.; Majeed, A.; Hayhoe, B. The impact of private online video consulting in primary care. *J. R. Soc. Med.* **2018**, *111*, 162–166. [CrossRef]
29. Han, S.M.; Greenfield, G.; Majeed, A.; Hayhoe, B. Impact of remote consultations on antibiotic prescribing in primary health care: Systematic review. *J. Med. Internet Res.* **2020**, *22*, 234–352. [CrossRef] [PubMed]
30. Hensey, C.C.; Gwee, A. Counterfeit drugs: An Australian perspective. *Med. J. Aust.* **2016**, *204*, 344–353. [CrossRef] [PubMed]
31. Hope, D.L.; Woods, P.; Mey, A.; Kelly, F.S.; Townshend, J.; Baumann-Birkbeck, L.M.; King, M.A. Australian pharmacists: Ready for increased non-prescription medicines reclassification. *Int. J. Pharm. Pract.* **2020**, *28*, 246–254. [CrossRef] [PubMed]
32. Mortazavi, S.S.; Shati, M.; Khankeh, H.R.; Ahmadi, F.; Mehravaran, S.; Malakouti, S.K. Self-medication among the elderly in Iran: A content analysis study. *BMC Geriatr.* **2017**, *17*, 198. [CrossRef]
33. Ajzen, I. The theory of planned behaviour: Frequently asked questions. *Hum. Behav. Emerg. Technol.* **2020**, *2*, 314–324. [CrossRef]
34. Ajzen, I. The theory of planned behaviour: Reactions and reflections. *Psychol. Health* **2011**, *26*, 1113–1127. [CrossRef]
35. Ajzen, I. The theory of planned behaviour. *Organ. Behav. Hum. Decis. Process.* **1991**, *50*, 179–211. [CrossRef]
36. La Barbera, F.; Ajzen, I. Control interactions in the theory of planned behavior: Rethinking the role of subjective norm. *Eur. J. Psychol.* **2020**, *16*, 401–417. [CrossRef]
37. Evans, I.E.M.; Martyr, A.; Collins, R.; Brayne, C.; Clare, L. Social isolation and cognitive function in later life: A systematic review and meta-analysis. *J. Alzheimer's Dis.* **2019**, *70*, 119–144. [CrossRef] [PubMed]
38. Gillis, C.; Mirzaei, F.; Potashman, M.; Ikram, M.A.; Maserejian, N. The incidence of mild cognitive impairment: A systematic review and data synthesis. *Alzheimer's Dement. Diagn. Assess. Dis. Monit.* **2019**, *11*, 248–256. [CrossRef] [PubMed]
39. John, A.; Patel, U.; Rusted, J.; Richards, M.; Gaysina, D. Affective problems and decline in cognitive state in older adults: A systematic review and meta-analysis. *Psychol. Med.* **2019**, *49*, 353–365. [CrossRef]
40. R Core Team. *R: A Language and Environment for Statistical Computing*; R Foundation for Statistical Computing: Vienna, Austria, 2022. Available online: https://www.R-project.org/ (accessed on 19 January 2023).
41. Project, T.J. Jamovi (Version 2.3.9.0) 2022. Available online: https://www.jamovi.org (accessed on 19 January 2023).
42. Reynolds, W.M. Development of reliable and valid short forms of the Marlowe-Crowne social desirability scale. *J. Clin. Psychol.* **1982**, *38*, 119–125. [CrossRef]
43. Kline, R.; Williams, M.; Vogt, W. Convergence of structural equation modeling and multilevel modeling. In *The SAGE Handbook of Innovation in Social Research Methods*; Sage Publications Ltd.: London, UK, 2011; pp. 562–603.
44. Palin, V.; Mölter, A.; Belmonte, M.; Ashcroft, D.M.; White, A.; Welfare, W.; van Staa, T. Antibiotic prescribing for common infections in UK general practice: Variability and drivers. *J. Antimicrob. Chemother.* **2019**, *74*, 2440–2450. [CrossRef]
45. Schröder, W.; Sommer, H.; Gladstone, B.P.; Foschi, F.; Hellman, J.; Evengard, B.; Tacconelli, E. Gender differences in antibiotic prescribing in the community: A systematic review and meta-analysis. *J. Antimicrob. Chemother.* **2016**, *71*, 1800–1806. [CrossRef] [PubMed]
46. Scaioli, G.; Gualano, M.R.; Gili, R.; Masucci, S.; Bert, F.; Siliquini, R. Antibiotic use: A cross-sectional survey assessing the knowledge, attitudes and practices amongst students of a school of medicine in Italy. *PLoS ONE* **2015**, *10*, 122–139. [CrossRef]
47. Fine, L.; Weinborn, M.; Ng, A.; Loft, S.; Li, Y.R.; Hodgson, E.; Parker, D.; Smith, S.R.; Sohrabi, H.R.; Brown, B.; et al. Sleep disruption explains age-related prospective memory deficits: Implications for cognitive aging and intervention. *Aging Neuropsychol. Cogn.* **2019**, *26*, 621–636. [CrossRef]
48. Lawrence, B.J.; Jayakody, D.M.P.; Bennett, R.J.; Eikelboom, R.H.; Gasson, N.; Friedland, P.L. Hearing loss and depression in older adults: A systematic review and meta-analysis. *Gerontologist* **2019**, *60*, 137–154. [CrossRef]
49. Scholes, G. Protein-energy malnutrition in older Australians: A narrative review of the prevalence, causes and consequences of malnutrition, and strategies for prevention. *Health Promot. J. Aust.* **2022**, *33*, 187–193. [CrossRef] [PubMed]
50. Lau, E.T.L.; Steadman, K.J.; Cichero, J.A.Y.; Nissen, L.M. Dosage form modification and oral drug delivery in older people. *Adv. Drug Deliv. Rev.* **2018**, *135*, 75–84. [CrossRef]
51. Hu, T.; Zhao, X.; Wu, M.; Li, Z.; Luo, L.; Yang, C.; Yang, F. Prevalence of depression in older adults: A systematic review and meta-analysis. *Psychiatry Res.* **2022**, *311*, 114–125. [CrossRef]
52. Lyons, A.; Alba, B.; Heywood, W.; Fileborn, B.; Minichiello, V.; Barrett, C.; Hinchliff, S.; Malta, S.; Dow, B. Experiences of ageism and the mental health of older adults. *Aging Ment. Health* **2018**, *22*, 1456–1464. [CrossRef]
53. Sussman, R.; Gifford, R. Causality in the theory of planned behavior. *Personal. Soc. Psychol. Bull.* **2019**, *45*, 920–933. [CrossRef]
54. Castanier, C.; Deroche, T.; Woodman, T. Theory of planned behaviour and road violations: The moderating influence of perceived behavioural control. *Transp. Res. Part F Traffic Psychol. Behav.* **2013**, *18*, 148–158. [CrossRef]
55. Poirier, G.; Ohayon, A.; Juranville, A.; Mourey, F.; Gaveau, J. Deterioration, compensation and motor control processes in healthy aging, mild cognitive impairment and Alzheimer's disease. *Geriatrics* **2021**, *6*, 33. [CrossRef] [PubMed]

56. Wildenbos, G.A.; Peute, L.; Jaspers, M. Aging barriers influencing mobile health usability for older adults: A literature based framework (MOLD-US). *Int. J. Med. Inform.* **2018**, *114*, 66–75. [CrossRef] [PubMed]
57. Lanz, L.; Thielmann, I.; Gerpott, F.H. Are social desirability scales desirable? A meta-analytic test of the validity of social desirability scales in the context of prosocial behavior. *J. Personal.* **2022**, *90*, 203–221. [CrossRef] [PubMed]
58. Chou, M.-Y.; Nishita, Y.; Nakagawa, T.; Tange, C.; Tomida, M.; Shimokata, H.; Otsuka, R.; Chen, L.-K.; Arai, H. Role of gait speed and grip strength in predicting 10-year cognitive decline among community-dwelling older people. *BMC Geriatr.* **2019**, *19*, 186. [CrossRef] [PubMed]
59. Holcombe, A.O.; Kovacs, M.; Aust, F.; Aczel, B. Documenting contributions to scholarly articles using CRediT and tenzing. *PLoS ONE* **2020**, *15*, e0244611. [CrossRef] [PubMed]

Disclaimer/Publisher's Note: The statements, opinions and data contained in all publications are solely those of the individual author(s) and contributor(s) and not of MDPI and/or the editor(s). MDPI and/or the editor(s) disclaim responsibility for any injury to people or property resulting from any ideas, methods, instructions or products referred to in the content.

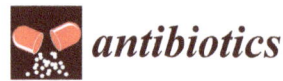

Article

A European International Multicentre Survey on the Current Practice of Perioperative Antibiotic Prophylaxis for Paediatric Liver Transplantations

Juliane Hauschild [1], Nora Bruns [1], Elke Lainka [2] and Christian Dohna-Schwake [1,*]

1 Department of Paediatrics I, University Hospital Essen, University of Duisburg-Essen, 45147 Essen, Germany
2 Department of Paediatrics II, University Hospital Essen, University of Duisburg-Essen, 45147 Essen, Germany
* Correspondence: christian.dohna-schwake@uk-essen.de

Abstract: (1) Background: Postoperative infections are major contributors of morbidity and mortality after paediatric liver transplantation (pLTX). Evidence and recommendations regarding the most effective antimicrobial strategy are lacking. (2) Results: Of 39 pLTX centres, 20 responded. Aminopenicillins plus ß-lactamase inhibitors were used by six (30%) and third generation cephalosporins by three (15%), with the remaining centres reporting heterogenous regimens. Broad-spectrum regimens were the standard in 10 (50%) of centres and less frequent in the 16 (80%) centres with an infectious disease specialist. The duration ranged mainly between 24–48 h and 3–5 days in the absence and 3–5 days or 6–10 days in the presence of risk factors. Strategies regarding antifungal, antiviral, adjunctive antimicrobial, and surveillance strategies varied widely. (3) Methods: This international multicentre survey endorsed by the European Liver Transplant Registry queried all European pLTX centres from the registry on their current practice of perioperative antibiotic prophylaxis and antimicrobial strategies via an online questionnaire. (4) Conclusions: This survey found great heterogeneity regarding all aspects of postoperative antimicrobial treatment, surveillance, and prevention of infections in European pLTX centres. Evidence-based recommendations are urgently needed to optimise antimicrobial strategies and reduce the spectrum and duration of antimicrobial exposure.

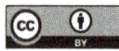

Keywords: paediatric liver transplantation; perioperative prophylaxis; antibiotics; antibiotic exposure; antimicrobials; infectious disease specialist; infection surveillance; infection prevention

1. Introduction

The first paediatric liver transplantations (pLTX) were performed in 1963, becoming the treatment of choice for acute and chronic liver diseases that cannot sufficiently be treated otherwise [1]. Today, the reported one-year survival exceeds 85% [2–4]. The remaining causes of morbidity and mortality in children mainly comprise early postoperative complications such as non- and poor-function of the liver, thrombosis of the portal vein or hepatic artery, haemorrhage and infections [5–7]. Forty-seven to 82% of these infections derive from bacterial origin [8–13] with long surgery times, transfusion of blood products, medical immunosuppression and disturbance of the mucosal gut barrier as the main risk factors. In a large registry study that included 2291 patients, 38% experienced a bacterial or fungal infection within 30 days after transplantation, and 5.5% died as a consequence of infection [14]. In a single centre study including 345 transplantations, 127 cases of sepsis, 22 cases of severe sepsis and 41 cases of septic shock were reported within the postoperative paediatric intensive care unit stay. Within this study population, septic shock was the leading cause of death [13,14].

Given the major influence of bacterial infections on the postoperative course after pLTX, the importance of effective preventive strategies seems under-represented in the literature and in guidelines. Perioperative antibiotic prophylaxis strategies as one example of prophylactic measure differ between centres [9,12,13,15–18]. It aims to prevent mainly surgical site infections and bacteraemia, but optimal choice of antimicrobial agent and length of therapy remains uncertain.

This study investigates the different anti-infective strategies and applications of antibiotics of European paediatric liver transplantation centres based on an online-survey, aiming to give an overview on anti-infective prevention measures.

2. Results

2.1. Demographics of Participating Centres

Out of 39 pLTX centres that were contacted, 23 (59%) questionnaires were answered, of which 20 (87%) met the eligibility criteria for analysis. The self-reported region of the participating centres was Western Europe (10/20; 50%), Central Europe (4/20; 20%), Northern Europe (3/20; 15%), Southern Europe (2/20; 10%), and Eastern Europe (1/20; 5%). Most participating centers performed more than 10 pLTXs including a few high urgency pLTXs and a varying number of living related pLTXs (Figure 1a–c). Immediate postoperative care was performed on paediatric and mixed intensive care units (16/20 (80%) and 4/20 (20%), respectively).

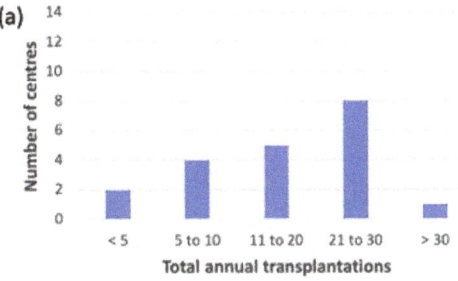

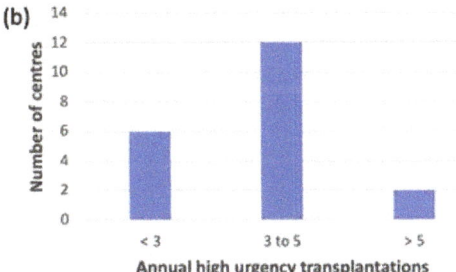

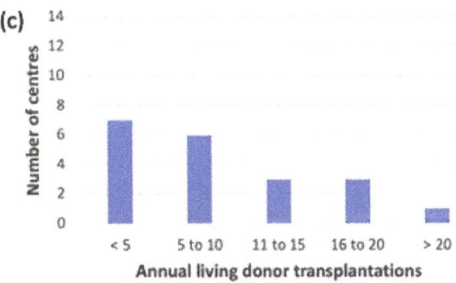

Figure 1. Annual frequency of paediatric liver transplantations in the participating centres. (a) Total number of annual transplantations. (b) Number of high urgency transplantations. (c) Living donor transplantations.

2.2. Immunosuppression

Seventeen (85%) centres used basiliximab for induction of immunosuppression. All centres included a calcineurin inhibitor (95% tacrolimus, 5% cyclosporine), and 13 (65%) centres used steroids as baseline immunosuppression with varying combinations of additional immunosuppressive substances (Table 1).

Table 1. Standard immunosuppression strategies in the first three weeks after paediatric liver transplantation in descending frequency.

n (%)	Steroid	Tacrolimus	CSA	MMF
10 (50%)	■	■		
6 (30%)	■	■		■
2 (10%)		■		■
1 (5%)	■		■	
1 (5%)		■	■	

CSA = Cyclosporine, MMF = mycophenolic mofetil. Grey boxes indicate the prescribed immunosuppression.

2.3. Antimicrobial Strategies

Standard perioperative antibiotic prophylaxis varied greatly, using an aminopenicillin plus beta lactamase inhibitor as most common choice (6/20; 30%) (Table 2). Eight centres (40%) used narrow spectrum antibiotics only, whereas 10 (50%) centres applied broad spectrum regimens. One centre reported that prophylaxis was tailored individually according to perioperative findings and another centre applied prophylaxis only to carriers of multidrug resistant bacteria. Antibiotics used to escalate treatment were mainly carbapenems, vancomycin, and ureidopenicillin plus beta lactamase inhibitor (Table 2).

The standard duration of antibiotic treatment varied across centres and was further adapted according to individual patients' risk factors (Figure 2). Fourteen centres (14/20; 70%) gave detailed information about the considered risk factors. These were MDR colonisation (9/14; 64%), presence of an abdominal patch (8/14; 57%), postoperative course of c-reactive protein levels (7/14; 50%), postoperative course of procalcitonin levels (6/14; 43%), antibiotic treatment prior to transplantation (6/14; 43%), pre-existing conditions (4/14; 29%), indwelling central lines (3/14; 21%), ascites after surgery (2/14; 14%), patient's age (1/14; 7%), length of hospitalisation prior to transplantation (1/14; 7%), and previous surgical procedures (1/14; 7%). When stratified for the annual number of transplantations, centres with lower numbers ($\leq$20) and centres with higher numbers of transplant patients (>20) showed similar duration of prophylaxis, but centres with lower numbers used a narrow spectrum antibiotic more often (Supplementary Table S1).

Antifungal prophylaxis in the absence specific risk factors was performed by 12 (60%) centres and included fluconazole, liposomal amphotericin B, micafungin, and caspofungin with varying risk factors triggering antifungal prophylaxis in the remaining centres (Supplementary Table S2). Cytomegalovirus (CMV) prophylaxis including aciclovir, ganciclovir or intravenous immunoglobulins was routinely administered to all patients in 7 of 17 (41%) centres and depended on additional risk factors in the remaining centres (Supplementary Table S2).

Infection surveillance strategies and non-pharmacological anti-infective measures varied greatly across centres (Supplementary Table S2). The majority of centres did not isolate the patients during the immediate postoperative course. Postoperative infectious management was mainly driven by teams of specialists that included a paediatric gastroenterologist in 14 (70%) centres, a paediatric infectious disease specialist in 10 (50%) centres, an infectious disease specialist in 6 (30%) centres, a paediatric intensive care specialist in 8 (40%) centres, a paediatric surgeon in 5 (25%) centres, an intensive care specialist in 3 (15%) centres, an anaesthetist in 2 (10%) centres and a surgeon, gastroenterologist or specialist for rational antibiotic therapy in one (5%) centre each.

Table 2. Antibiotics for perioperative prophylaxis and for escalation therapy.

n (%)	Narrow Spectrum			Broad Spectrum								
	1st gen. Cephalosporin	Amino-Penicillin	Amino-Penicillin + BLI	3rd gen. Cephalosporin	4th gen. Cephalosporin	Ureidopenicillin + BLI	Carbapenem	Fluoroquinolone	Glycopeptide	Amino-Glycoside	Colistin	Tigecycline
6 (30%)			Green									
3 (15%)		Grey		Grey								
2 (10%)		Green										
1 (5%)				Grey								
2 (10%)			Grey			Grey						
1 (5%)	Green											
1 (5%)							Grey	Grey				
17 (85%)										Grey		
7 (35%)									Blue			
5 (25%)						Blue	Blue					
1 (5%)					Blue							
2 (10%)									Blue			
2 (10%)								Blue				
1 (5%)												
1 (5%)											Blue	
1 (5%)												Blue

Green = use of narrow spectrum antibiotics only. Blue = Antibiotics used for escalation of treatment. Grey = use of either narrow and broad spectrum antibiotics or broad spectrum antibiotics only. BLI = Beta-lactamase inhibitor; gen. = generation.

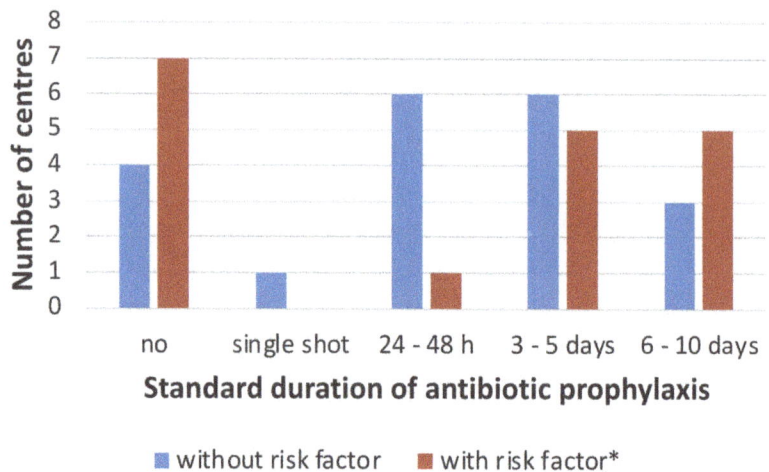

Figure 2. Duration of perioperative antibiotic prophylaxis, and according to additional risk factors in paediatric liver transplantation recipients. * Risk factors: defined by the treating physician/team, e.g., length of hospital stay, antibiotic treatment or intra-abdominal patch.

2.4. MDR Prevalence and Perioperative Prophylaxis

The prevalence of MDR bacteria was low in the majority of centres (Supplementary Figure S1). Among MRSA low prevalence-centres, 7 (69%) applied broad-spectrum antibiotics as prophylaxis (Table 3). The duration of prophylaxis ranged between 3–5 days in four of these centres and between 24–48 h in three centres. All centres with high MRSA prevalence used narrow-spectrum antibiotic prophylaxis.

Table 3. Association of prophylaxis spectrum with prevalence of multidrug resistance and availability of infectious disease specialists.

		n (%)	Narrow-Spectrum Prophylaxis n (%)	Broad-Spectrum Prophylaxis n (%)
(Paediatric) infectious disease specialist	Yes	16 (80%)	9 (56%)	7 (44%)
	No	4 (20%)	1 (25%)	3 (75%)
MRSA prevalence *	Low (<5%)	11 (69%)	4 (36%)	7 (64%)
	High (≥5%)	5 (31%)	5 (100%)	0 (0%)
ESBL prevalence *	Low (<20%)	10 (63%)	8 (80%)	2 (20%)
	High (≥20%)	6 (38%)	1 (17%)	5 (63%)

* Total number of answers n = 16.

In the majority of centres with low ESBL prevalence (<20%) a narrow-spectrum prophylaxis (8 centres, 80%) was prescribed. The duration of the prophylaxis was limited to 24–48 h in four of these centres. Five of six centres with high ESBL prevalence used broad-spectrum antibiotics instead. Three of these centres limited the duration of the prophylaxis to 3–5 days.

2.5. Availability of a (Paediatric) Infectious Disease Specialist and Perioperative Prophylaxis

Nine (56%) centres with involvement of an infectious disease specialist used narrow-spectrum antibiotics as prophylaxis. The duration of prophylaxis was limited to either 24–48 h or 3–5 days in 31.3% of the cases, respectively. Of the four centres without infectious disease specialist, three used broad-spectrum prophylaxis.

3. Discussion

Children in the early phase after liver transplantation are at an increased risk for an infection, but evidence on optimal prevention strategies and current practice is limited. The results of this survey present an overview of anti-infective prevention strategies with a focus on perioperative antibiotic prophylaxis used in 20 pLTX centres across Europe. We observed striking differences between the centres especially regarding the choice and duration of antibiotic application. For example, the duration of perioperative prophylaxis ranged between an intraoperative single shot and 6–10 days. Similar differences were reported for antifungal, antiviral, non-pharmacological anti-infective measures and surveillance strategies.

The observed differences reflect the under-represented topic of infection control and especially perioperative antimicrobial prophylaxis in the current literature. Reviews and state-of-the-art articles on paediatric liver transplantation neither include abstracts about infection control measures nor give any recommendations [19,20]. In a book chapter on early post-transplant management duration of postoperative prophylaxis is given for 5 days, either cefuroxime or cefazoline [21].

In the absence of guidelines or recommendations, the observed differences might be explained in part by centre specifics like prevalence of MDR pathogens, availability of infectious disease specialists and the clinical experience of the staff taking care of children after transplantation. Nevertheless, most centres in our study used longer antibiotic prophylaxis than the recommended standard in most of other major surgeries. This corresponds to the results of previous point prevalence studies, which reported prolonged antibiotic courses in critically ill children [22] and prolonged postoperative prophylaxis rates after major surgeries of up to 87% [23]. In this context, it seems necessary to point out that the potential harm of antibiotic is vast and must indispensably be outweighed against the potential benefits [24].

Very likely, the potential of reducing exposure to antimicrobial substances is not fully exploited. Early infectious complications after pLTX occurred in about 50% of cases in patients with antibiotic prophylaxis duration <48 h [12,13] and ≥48 h [9,15,16]. A pre-post design study on the implementation of standardized postoperative antimicrobial prophylaxis after pLTX achieved a reduction of broad-spectrum antibiotics covering mainly gram-negative bacteria for more than 48 h post-op from 77% to 44% and vancomycin use from 50% to 7% without an increase in adverse events [18]. As surgical site infection is one of the major contributors to complications in the early phase after pLTX, high quality prospective studies are needed to collect further evidence on the optimal duration of perioperative prophylaxis in order to optimize treatment effects and reduce harm from inadequate antibiotic exposure. Possibly, non-pharmacological or intraoperative measures and the improvement of surgery results carry the potential to further reduce surgical site infections [25].

Another striking heterogeneity of our survey was the choice of antibiotic substances used for perioperative prophylaxis. In the literature, similar heterogeneity has been reported with regimens ranging from carboxypenicillin plus ß-lactamase inhibitor to aminopenicillins plus third generation cephalosporins with or without metronidazole to ureidopenicillin plus ß-lactamase inhibitor with or without aminoglycoside [9,12,13,15–18]. In all cited studies, the rate of postoperative infections was reported at around 50%. The results of these studies suggest that the impact of specific antibiotic regimens on the development of postoperative infections after pLTX is limited. This limited impact may partially explain the different strategies between centres and at the same time carries the potential to optimise perioperative prophylaxis by narrowing the spectrum and duration of administered antibiotics to an acceptable minimum.

An important barrier to narrowing the spectrum of perioperative prophylaxis after pLTX are MDR bacteria, as these pathogens constitute a clinically relevant cause of postoperative infections, sepsis, and septic shock [3,8,12,13,16,18]. The participants of our survey stated that they adapted antibiotic strategies according to the presence of MDR bacteria—centres with high prevalence of ESBL pathogens reported broader-spectrum regimens than low prevalence-centres. Apparently, prophylactic regimens are adapted according to local epidemiological considerations, which should also be taken into account when developing guidelines or recommendations in the future. Possibly, individually tailored perioperative prophylaxis is needed in MDR carriers.

Another factor that potentially influences the incidence and course of postoperative and surgical site infections in pLTX patients is the integration of infectious disease specialists in postoperative antimicrobial management. In this survey, 80% of the centres reported that they had support by infectious disease specialists. These centres were less likely to use broad-spectrum perioperative prophylaxis. Alongside optimised prescription of antimicrobials, further non-pharmacological measures of surveillance and prevention may play a role, such as routine cultures and swabs, isolation, and local antiseptic measures. The answers from our survey yielded great heterogeneity regarding these measures. In future prospective studies in the field of infectious complications after pLTX, these factors should be harmonized in order to rule them out as confounding effects of these measures and, if possible, gather evidence on their effectiveness.

The major limitation of our study is the small number of participants, limiting in depth analyses on associations between different hospital characteristics and parameters of interest. Further, the survey was conducted anonymously with the self-reported region as only indicator of the geographical distribution of participating centres. This limitation is especially important to highlight as the prevalence of MDR bacteria varies very much across the regions, for ESBL from almost zero in Scandinavia to much higher percentages in Southern European countries [26]. Due to the anonymity, we cannot rule out double participation of a centre, even though we did not find duplicate answer profiles and no double naming of a hospital in the voluntary question.

Nonetheless, this survey is an important contribution to understanding the current practice of perioperative antibiotic prophylaxis in Europe. The diversity of antibiotic and antimicrobial strategies and duration of prophylaxis we found is likely caused by local epidemiologic situations regarding MDR prevalence and further promoted by the lack of evidence-based recommendations. The availability of infectious disease specialists seems to foster narrow-spectrum perioperative prophylaxis, whereas high prevalence of ESBL pathogens was associated with broad-spectrum prophylaxis. The need to reduce harm from unwarranted, too long or too broad antibiotic treatment for the individual pLTX patient, critically ill children, and for society in general is high. This implies that prospective randomized controlled trials on the minimally necessary duration of perioperative prophylaxis, adequate substances, and effective additional measures after pLTX are urgently needed in order to optimise postoperative infectious care of these vulnerable patients.

4. Materials and Methods

4.1. Study Design

The official contact persons of paediatric liver transplantation centres participating in the European Liver Transplant Registry (ELTR) were queried via email to answer an online survey (SurveyMonkey®) in December 2020 and in July 2021. Additionally, some centres were contacted personally by using official contact addresses from the hospitals' websites. All questionnaires were filled in anonymously by the contact person from each centre with voluntary naming of the respective hospital.

The questionnaire was based on personal experience and the study of Vandecasteele on antimicrobial prophylaxis in adult liver transplantation [27]. It was reviewed, endorsed, and officially promoted by the ELTR. The questionnaire consisted of 30 questions including (i) the standard duration and type of antibiotic prophylaxis, the duration in patients with high risk for infection, and antibiotic choices in case of escalation, (ii) the annual number of total paediatric liver transplantations, living donor and high-urgency liver transplantations, (iii) the prevalence of multi-drug resistant bacteria (MDR), availability of infectious disease specialists, (iv) the strategies of immunosuppression, perioperative care and antiseptic measures, and (v) prophylactic antifungal and antiviral therapies (Supplementary File).

4.2. Data Analysis

Only questionnaires with at least the first four questions answered were eligible for analysis. Data are summarized as counts and frequencies. Because not all questions were answered by all participants, the denominator may vary and for that reason is given for each individual item. Some answers were categorized, e.g., the number of transplantations per year. All statistical analyses were performed with IBM SPSS Statistic for Windows, version 27 (Armonk, NY, USA). Figures were produced using Microsoft Office Excel for Mac Version 16.65 (Microsoft Corporation, Redmont, WA, USA).

4.3. Ethics Approval and Support

The European Liver Transplant Registry approved and supported the survey (acceptance letter 6 October 2020). The ethic committee of the medical faculty of Duisburg-Essen waived the need for ethic approval because no patient data were involved.

5. Conclusions

To conclude, this survey is the first to give an overview on current perioperative antibiotic prophylaxis after paediatric liver transplantation in Europe. We report inter-centre heterogeneity regarding all aspects of postoperative antimicrobial treatment, surveillance, and prevention of infections. The involvement of infectious disease specialists in postoperative management of infections was widespread and was associated with a higher proportion of narrow-spectrum perioperative prophylaxis. The results from this study imply that evidence-based recommendations are urgently needed in order to optimise pharmacological and non-pharmacological antimicrobial strategies and reduce exposure antimicrobials to the necessary minimum in terms of duration and spectrum.

Supplementary Materials: The following supporting information can be downloaded at: https://www.mdpi.com/article/10.3390/antibiotics12020292/s1, Figure S1: Prevalence of multidrug resistant bacteria in participating paediatric liver transplantation centres; Table S1: Duration and type of antibiotic prophylaxis according to the number of annual transplantations; Table S2: Infection surveillance strategies and non-antibiotic anti-infective measures.

Author Contributions: Conceptualization, J.H. and C.D.-S.; methodology, J.H., N.B. and C.D.-S.; software, J.H., N.B. and C.D.-S.; validation, J.H., N.B. and C.D.-S.; formal analysis, J.H., N.B. and C.D.-S.; investigation, J.H., N.B. and C.D.-S.; resources, J.H. and C.D.-S.; data curation, J.H., N.B. and C.D.-S.; writing—original draft preparation, J.H.; writing—review and editing N.B., C.D.-S. and E.L.; visualization, J.H. and N.B.; supervision, C.D.-S.; project administration, C.D.-S. All authors have read and agreed to the published version of the manuscript.

Funding: No funding was received for the study.

Institutional Review Board Statement: The ethic committee of the Medical Faculty of Duisburg-Essen waived the need for ethic approval because no patient data were involved.

Informed Consent Statement: No patients were involved in the study.

Data Availability Statement: Data will be made available to any qualified researcher without undue reservation upon reasonable request.

Acknowledgments: We would like to thank the participants of this survey for their contributions.

Conflicts of Interest: The authors declare no conflict of interest.

References

1. Starzl, T.E.; Groth, C.G.; Brettschneider, L.; Penn, I.; Fulginiti, V.A.; Moon, J.B.; Blanchard, H.; Martin, A.J.; Porter, K.A. Orthotopic Homotransplantation of the Human Liver. *Ann. Surg.* **1968**, *168*, 392–415. [CrossRef]
2. Basturk, A.; Yılmaz, A.; Sayar, E.; Dinçkan, A.; Aliosmanoğlu, İ.; Erbiş, H.; Aydınlı, B.; Artan, R. Pediatric Liver Transplantation: Our Experiences. *Eurasian J. Med.* **2016**, *48*, 209–212. [CrossRef]
3. Pfister, E.-D. 40 Jahre Lebertransplantation im Kindes- und Jugendalter. *Mon. Kinderheilkd.* **2016**, *164*, 455–464. [CrossRef]
4. Sundaram, S.S.; Alonso, E.M.; Anand, R.; Study of Pediatric Liver Transplantation Research Group. Outcomes after liver transplantation in young infants. *J. Pediatr. Gastroenterol. Nutr.* **2008**, *47*, 486–492. [CrossRef]
5. Cacciarelli, T.V.; Dvorchik, I.; Mazariegos, G.V.; Gerber, D.; Jain, A.B.; Fung, J.J.; Reyes, J. An analysis of pretransplantation variables associated with long-term allograft outcome in pediatric liver transplant recipients receiving primary tacrolimus (FK506) therapy. *Transplantation* **1999**, *68*, 650–655. [CrossRef]
6. Saint-Vil, D.; Luks, F.I.; Lebel, P.; Brandt, M.L.; Paradis, K.; Weber, A.; Guay, J.; Guttman, F.M.; Bensoussan, A.; Laberge, J.-M.; et al. Infectious complications of pediatric liver transplantation. *J. Pediatr. Surg.* **1991**, *26*, 908–913. [CrossRef]
7. Van Heerden, Y.; Maher, H.; Etheredge, H.; Fabian, J.; Grieve, A.; Loveland, J.; Botha, J. Outcomes of paediatric liver transplant for biliary atresia. *S. Afr. J. Surg.* **2019**, *57*, 17–23. [CrossRef]
8. Alcamo, A.M.; Alessi, L.J.; Vehovic, S.N.; Bansal, N.; Bond, G.J.; Carcillo, J.A.; Green, M.; Michaels, M.G.; Aneja, R.K. Severe Sepsis in Pediatric Liver Transplant Patients: The Emergence of Multidrug-Resistant Organisms. *Pediatr. Crit. Care Med.* **2019**, *20*, e326–e332. [CrossRef]
9. Ashkenazi-Hoffnung, L.; Mozer-Glassberg, Y.; Bilavsky, E.; Yassin, R.; Shamir, R.; Amir, J. Children Post Liver Trans-plantation Hospitalized with Fever Are at a High Risk for Bacterial Infections. *Transpl. Infect. Dis.* **2016**, *18*, 333–340. [CrossRef]
10. Bouchut, J.-C.; Stamm, D.; Boillot, O.; Lepape, A.; Floret, D. Postoperative infectious complications in paediatric liver transplantation: A study of 48 transplants. *Pediatr. Anesth.* **2001**, *11*, 93–98. [CrossRef]
11. Kim, J.C.; Lee, J.K.; Yang, S.I.; Park, S.H.; Yoon, K.W.; Lee, H.; Yi, N.J.; Suh, K.S.; Choi, E.H.; Lee, H.J. Incidence and Risk Factors for Infections After Liver Transplant in Children: Single-Center Experience for 15 Years. *Open Forum Infect. Dis.* **2017**, *4*, S704. [CrossRef]
12. Béranger, A.; Capito, C.; Lacaille, F.; Ferroni, A.; Bouazza, N.; Girard, M.; Oualha, M.; Renolleau, S.; Debray, D.; Chardot, C.; et al. Early Bacterial Infections after Pediatric Liver Transplantation in the Era of Multidrug-Resistant Bacteria: Nine-Year Single-Center Retrospective Experience. *Pediatr. Infect. Dis. J.* **2020**, *39*, e169–e175. [CrossRef]
13. Schwake, C.D.; Guiddir, T.; Cuzon, G.; Benissa, M.-R.; Dubois, C.; Miatello, J.; Merchaoui, Z.; Durand, P.; Tissieres, P. For the Bicêtre Pediatric Liver Transplant Group Bacterial infections in children after liver transplantation: A single-center surveillance study of 345 consecutive transplantations. *Transpl. Infect. Dis.* **2019**, *22*, e13208. [CrossRef]
14. Shepherd, R.W.; Turmelle, Y.; Nadler, M.; Lowell, J.A.; Narkewicz, M.R.; McDiarmid, S.V.; Anand, R.; Song, C. Risk Factors for Rejection and Infection in Pediatric Liver Transplantation. *Am. J. Transplant.* **2007**, *8*, 396–403. [CrossRef] [PubMed]
15. Ganschow, R.; Nolkemper, D.; Helmke, K.; Harps, E.; Commentz, J.C.; Broering, D.C.; Pothmann, W.; Rogiers, X.; Hellwege, H.H.; Burdelski, M. Intensive Care Management after Pediatric Liver Transplantation: A Single-Center Expe-rience. *Pediatr. Transplant.* **2000**, *4*, 273–279. [CrossRef]
16. Phichaphop, C.; Apiwattanakul, N.; Techasaensiri, C.; Lertudomphonwanit, C.; Treepongkaruna, S.; Thirapattaraphan, C.; Boonsathorn, S. High prevalence of multidrug-resistant gram-negative bacterial infection following pediatric liver transplantation. *Medicine* **2020**, *99*, e23169. [CrossRef]
17. Uemoto, S.; Tanaka, K.; Fujita, S.; Sano, K.; Shirahase, I.; Kato, H.; Yamamoto, E.; Inomata, Y.; Ozawa, K. Infectious complications in living related liver transplantation. *J. Pediatr. Surg.* **1994**, *29*, 514–517. [CrossRef]
18. Bio, L.L.; Schwenk, H.T.; Chen, S.F.; Conlon, S.; Gallo, A.; Bonham, C.A.; Gans, H.A. Standardization of Post-Operative Antimicrobials Reduced Exposure While Maintaining Good Outcomes in Pediatric Liver Transplant Recipients. *Transpl. Infect. Dis.* **2021**, *23*, e13538. [CrossRef]
19. Kohli, R.; Cortes, M.; Heaton, N.D.; Dhawan, A. Liver transplantation in children: State of the art and future persoectives. *Arch. Dis. Child.* **2018**, *103*, 192–198. [CrossRef]
20. Pham, Y.H.; Miloh, T. Liver transplantation in children. *Clin. Liver. Dis.* **2018**, *22*, 807–821. [CrossRef]
21. Rock, N.M.; McLin, V.A. Listing for Transplantation; Postoperative Management and Long-Term Follow-Up. In *Pediatric Hepatology and Liver Transplantation*; D'Antiga, L., Ed.; Springer: Berlin/Heidelberg, Germany, 2019; pp. 515–534.
22. Noël, K.C.; Papenburg, J.; Lacroix, J.; Quach, C.; O'Donnell, S.; Gonzales, M.; Willson, D.F.; Gilfoyle, E.; McNally, J.D.; Reynolds, S.; et al. International Survey on Determinants of Antibiotic Duration and Discontinuation in Pediatric Critically Ill Patients. *Pediatr. Crit. Care Med.* **2020**, *21*, e696–e704. [CrossRef]
23. Versporten, A.; Bielicki, J.; Drapier, N.; Sharland, M.; Goossens, H.; ARPEC Project Group; Calle, G.M.; Garrahan, J.P.; Clark, J.; Cooper, C.; et al. The Worldwide Antibiotic Resistance and Prescribing in European Children (ARPEC) point prevalence survey: Developing hospital-quality indicators of antibiotic prescribing for children. *J. Antimicrob. Chemother.* **2016**, *71*, 1106–1117. [CrossRef]
24. Bruns, N.; Dohna-Schwake, C. Antibiotics in critically ill children—A narrative review on different aspects of a rational approach. *Pediatr. Res.* **2021**, *91*, 440–446. [CrossRef]

25. Hollenbeak, C.S.; Alfrey, E.J.; Sheridan, K.; Burger, T.L.; Dillon, P.W. Surgical site infections following pediatric liver transplantation: Risks and costs. *Transpl. Infect. Dis.* **2003**, *5*, 72–78. [CrossRef]
26. Antimicrobial Rsistance Collaborators. Global burden of bacterial antimicrobial resistance in 2019: A systematic analysis. *Lancet* **2022**, *399*, 629–655. [CrossRef]
27. Vandecasteele, E.; De Waele, J.; Vandijck, D.; Blot, S.; Vogelaers, D.; Rogiers, X.; Van Vlierberghe, H.; Decruyenaere, J.; Hoste, E. Antimicrobial prophylaxis in liver transplant patients—A multicenter survey endorsed by the European Liver and Intestine Transplant Association. *Transpl. Int.* **2009**, *23*, 182–190. [CrossRef]

Disclaimer/Publisher's Note: The statements, opinions and data contained in all publications are solely those of the individual author(s) and contributor(s) and not of MDPI and/or the editor(s). MDPI and/or the editor(s) disclaim responsibility for any injury to people or property resulting from any ideas, methods, instructions or products referred to in the content.

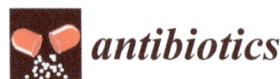

Article

Developing a Tool for Auditing the Quality of Antibiotic Dispensing in Community Pharmacies: A Pilot Study

Maarten Lambert [1,*], Ria Benkő [2], Athina Chalkidou [3], Jesper Lykkegaard [4], Malene Plejdrup Hansen [4,5], Carl Llor [6], Pia Touboul [7], Indrė Trečiokienė [1,8], Maria-Nefeli Karkana [9], Anna Kowalczyk [10] and Katja Taxis [1]

1. Unit of PharmacoTherapy, Epidemiology and Economics, Groningen Research Institute of Pharmacy, University of Groningen, 9713 AV Groningen, The Netherlands
2. Department of Clinical Pharmacy and Albert Szent-Györgyi Medical Center, Central Pharmacy and Emergency Care Department, University of Szeged, 6720 Szeged, Hungary
3. Section of General Practice, Department of Public Health, University of Copenhagen, 1353 Copenhagen, Denmark
4. Audit Project Odense, Research Unit of General Practice, University of Southern Denmark, 5230 Odense, Denmark
5. Center for General Practice, Aalborg University, 9220 Aalborg, Denmark
6. Institut Català de la Salut, Via Roma Health Centre, 08007 Barcelona, Spain
7. Department of Public Health, Nice University Hospital, 06202 Nice, France
8. Institute of Biomedical Sciences, Faculty of Medicine, Pharmacy Center, Vilnius University, 03101 Vilnius, Lithuania
9. Clinic of Social and Family Medicine, Faculty of Medicine, University of Crete, 71003 Heraklion, Crete, Greece
10. Centre for Family and Community Medicine, Faculty of Health Sciences, Medical University of Lodz, 90-153 Lodz, Poland
* Correspondence: m.lambert@rug.nl; Tel.: +316-29102971

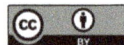

Abstract: Background: The European Centre for Disease Prevention and Control describes the community pharmacist as the gatekeeper to the quality of antibiotic use. The pharmacist has the responsibility to guard safe and effective antibiotic use; however, little is known about how this is implemented in practice. Aims: To assess the feasibility of a method to audit the quality of antibiotic dispensing in community pharmacy practice and to explore antibiotic dispensing practices in Greece, Lithuania, Poland, and Spain. Methods: The Audit Project Odense methodology to audit antibiotic dispensing practice was adapted for use in community pharmacy practice. Community pharmacists registered antibiotic dispensing on a specifically developed registration chart and were asked to provide feedback on the registration method. Results: Altogether, twenty pharmacists were recruited in four countries. They registered a total of 409 dispenses of oral antibiotics. Generally, pharmacists were positive about the feasibility of implementing the registration chart in practice. The frequency of checking for allergies, contraindications and interactions differed largely between the four countries. Pharmacists provided little advice to patients. The pharmacists rarely contacted prescribers. Conclusion: This tool seems to make it possible to get a useful picture of antibiotic dispensing patterns in community pharmacies. Dispensing practice does not seem to correspond with EU guidelines according to these preliminary results.

Keywords: community pharmacy practice; dispensing quality; antibiotics; antimicrobial resistance; Audit Project Odense

1. Introduction

Community pharmacists are in a unique position to positively impact antibiotic use and reduce antimicrobial resistance [1,2]. The European Centre for Disease Prevention and Control (ECDC) has established guidelines for the prudent use of antimicrobials for human consumption, explicitly stating that community pharmacists are gatekeepers to antibiotic use [3]. As gatekeepers, community pharmacists can reduce unnecessary antibiotic use for self-limiting infections and ensure optimal use of antibiotics [3]. In this role, pharmacists act as a source of information for patients and prescribers on the safe, rational, and effective use of antimicrobials [3]. This includes a responsibility to dispense antibiotics based on valid prescriptions which includes checking the rationale for treatment, providing advice, and performing safety checks of contraindications and interactions [3]. Correspondingly, the World Health Organization (WHO) and the International Pharmaceutical Federation have developed guidelines for good pharmacy practice, emphasizing similar responsibilities for community pharmacists [4,5]. Consequently, these organizations advocate the key role that community pharmacists should play in addressing the problem of antimicrobial resistance.

Currently, little is known about dispensing practices for antibiotics in community pharmacies and to what extent pharmacists fulfil the role as gatekeeper to antibiotic use in daily practice. In their systematic review on documenting dispensing practices [6], Cerqueira-Santos et al. stress the need for novel strategies to document the dispensing process to ensure better pharmacy practice with regard to patients and other healthcare professionals. Moreover, as dispensing practices are likely to differ between drug classes, such documenting strategies are preferably specifically adjusted to different drug classes. In order to map antibiotic dispensing practices and gain insight to what extent community pharmacists adhere to current EU guidelines, a specific tool is needed for documenting antibiotic dispensing, as such a tool does not exist yet. Ideally, such a tool must be easy to implement in daily practice and quick to use.

The Audit Project Odense Methodology

One way to document healthcare practice is through self-registry by healthcare professionals. In general practice for example, the Audit Project Odense (APO) methodology was developed for quality improvement [7] and is used to successfully decrease inappropriate use of antibiotics [8]. The APO method encompasses a bottom-up approach to implement multi-faceted interventions. The core components of this method are two audit registrations [9]. General practitioners register key variables about diagnosis of infectious diseases and prescribing of antibiotics on a pre-specified chart, including patient symptoms, diagnostics, and choice of treatment. In the community pharmacy setting, the APO methodology has not been used previously. Based on the promising results in general practice, applying the APO methodology in the community pharmacy practice setting may be an innovative way to improve antibiotic use through documenting dispensing practices. Therefore, this paper describes the development and pilot testing of an audit chart in the community pharmacy setting. Specifically, the aims of the pilot study are three-fold:

1. To assess the feasibility of registering antibiotic dispensing using the registration chart in the community pharmacy setting;
2. To collect feedback from community pharmacists on the implementation of the APO method;
3. To describe antibiotic dispensing practices in four European countries.

2. Results

2.1. Feasibility of the APO-Methodology in Community Pharmacy Practice

In total, 20 pharmacies were recruited to participate in the pilot study, five in each of the four countries. One pharmacy in Greece dropped out of the study due to intense workload. All participants ($n = 19$) returned the questionnaire. The participation of pharmacy staff differed between the pharmacies. In 10 pharmacies, both pharmacists and pharmacist technicians participated in the pilot study. In four pharmacies, only one staff member participated; this could either be a pharmacist or a pharmacist technician. In three pharmacies, more than one staff member participated, although not the entire staff. In the remaining two pharmacies, only pharmacists participated. All pharmacies reported that registration of patients took less than one minute per dispensed antibiotic or between one and two minutes, except for one pharmacy that needed two to three minutes per registration. In all countries, pharmacy staff managed to register all patients with a prescription for an oral antibiotic or only missed a couple of dispenses during the study period. Reasons for not registering included high workload or forgetting. Most of the pharmacists found the registration chart, instruction form, and list of antibiotics clear and easy to use.

2.2. Antibiotic Dispensing Practice

During the study period, a total of 409 dispenses of antibiotics were registered. Of those antibiotics, 59% were prescribed to female patients, with the average patient age being 43 years (SD = 24 years). The most frequently dispensed antibiotics were amoxicillin and amoxicillin/clavulanic acid, followed by macrolides or clindamycin and cephalosporines, although frequencies differed per country. In total, 77% of the dispenses were registered by pharmacists, 22% by other pharmacy staff, in 2% this was not reported. Nearly half of the dispensed antibiotics were prescribed for acute respiratory tract infections. The indication for the prescribed antibiotic was unknown to the pharmacy staff for 11% of the total number of dispenses. There was contact between the pharmacist and the prescriber for 14 (3%) of the dispenses, which led to changes to the prescription in nine (2%) cases. In Poland, there was no contact with prescribers at all, and in 12% of the dispenses this information was not reported (Table 1).

The frequency of checking for drug-drug interactions, contraindications, and allergies during the dispensing process differed largely between the countries. In total, in 49% of the dispenses none of the three safety checks were performed. However, in 70% of the cases in Lithuania none of the checks were performed, whereas in Greece no checks were performed in 18% of the cases. When looking at the individual safety checks, checking for contraindications was performed the least often (21%) and checking for allergies most often (36%). Only in Spain and Greece were there dispenses for which all three safety checks were performed, in 24% and 22% of registrations, respectively (Table 1).

Overall, in 66% of the dispenses, the pharmacy staff discussed treatment duration with patients. Other general advice that is deemed appropriate to give during dispensing of all antibiotics was given less frequently: information about side effects (21%), informing about risk of AMR (18%), seeking medical help if symptoms worsen (19%), and bringing back leftovers (4%). In 13% of the dispenses, the pharmacist did not provide the patient with any advice (Appendix A).

Treatment duration was unknown for 7% of the dispensed antibiotics. In 70% of the dispenses, the pharmacy staff deemed the prescription appropriate for the specific situation on a clinical basis (e.g., necessity of antibiotic, correct choice of antibiotic, correct dose, correct treatment duration), in 3% the pharmacy staff did not agree, and in 26% the staff reported to not have sufficient information to make this judgement. This information was missing in 1%. In 31 cases, pharmacists judged a prescription as appropriate despite not knowing the indication and/or treatment duration, which was considered as inappropriate agreement (Appendix A). Four antibiotics were dispensed after wait-and-see advice from the prescriber.

2.3. Feedback on the Registration Chart

Most feedback was about the domain of advice on the registration chart and instruction form. For example, for "discuss treatment duration" one Spanish pharmacist commented: 'does this mean to explain and reinforce the importance of not stopping treatment until finishing it, or only explain the duration of treatment?'. Moreover, pharmacists reported they found some advice unnecessary to give while missing other information, although this feedback differed per pharmacy, within and between the countries. Several other topics were suggested to be added to the registration chart, including veterinarian use, probiotics, prophylaxis, injectable antibiotics, metronidazole, treatment preparation, and storage.

Table 1. Characteristics of registered dispenses.

	Greece	Lithuania	Poland	Spain	Total	Total (%)	Missing
Dispenses registered	55 (13.4%)	103 (25.2%)	74 (18.1%)	177 (43.3%)	409	100	
Sex							0 (0%)
Female	32	69	42	97	240	58.7	
Male	23	34	32	80	169	41.3	
Education							7 (1.7%)
Pharmacist	38	92	68	116	314	76.8	
Not pharmacist	17	8	6	57	88	21.5	
Antibiotics dispensed							2 (0.5%)
Penicillin V or pivmecillinam	0	0	2	2	4	1.0	
Amoxicillin	7	20	6	36	69	16.9	
Amoxicillin + clavulanic acid	17	25	13	31	86	21.0	
Fosfomycin	0	1	1	29	31	7.6	
Nitrofurantoin	0	10	1	2	13	3.2	
Trimethoprim +/− Sulphonamides	0	4	2	1	7	1.7	
Macrolides or clindamycin	1	9	26	31	67	16.4	
Tetracyclines	2	9	4	2	17	4.2	
Cephalosporins	11	12	10	16	49	12.0	
Quinolones	12	2	5	19	38	9.3	
Other	5	9	4	8	26	6.4	
Focus of infection							1 (0.2%)
Respiratory tract	28	42	52	80	202	49.4	
Urinary tract	7	16	6	45	74	18.1	
Gastrointestinal	6	4	1	11	22	5.4	
Skin	2	1	5	11	19	4.7	
Gynaecological	1	1	1	0	3	0.7	
Other	9	10	1	23	43	10.5	
Unknown	2	29	8	6	45	11.0	
Safety checks performed							
Interactions	25	10	23	58	116	28.4	
Contraindications	20	1	8	55	84	20.5	
Allergies	38	16	15	78	147	35.9	
None of the above	10	72	38	82	202	49.4	
All safety checks performed	12	0	0	42	54	13.2	
Prescriber contact							49 (12.0%)
Yes, and changes to prescription	0	8	0	1	9	2.2	
Yes, no changes to prescription	2	0	0	3	5	1.2	
No contact with prescriber	34	89	74	149	346	84.6	
Pharmacy judgement of prescription							2 (0.5%)
Agree with prescription	39	86	51	110	286	69.9	
Do not agree with prescription	5	3	0	6	14	3.4	
Insufficient information to decide	10	13	23	61	107	26.2	

Similarly, suggestions were provided for changes to other domains of the registration chart. Pharmacists in Greece described that it was difficult and uncommon to contact prescribers. In Lithuania, pharmacists reported that most of the time it was almost impossible to contact prescribers for clarification or changes to the prescription. Interestingly, the registrations during the pilot study show that in Greece there was contact with the prescriber in 5.5% of the cases and in Lithuania in 8.2% of the cases, whereas in Poland this was 0%. Additionally, some Lithuanian pharmacists mentioned that safety checks for contraindications and interactions were not performed in their pharmacies and patients were usually not informed about side effects from drug use. This aligns with the registered dispenses, as contraindications were only checked in 1.0% of cases, interactions, and allergies in 9.7% and 15.5%, respectively, and information about side effects was provided in 2.9% of the dispenses. Polish pharmacists reported that it was often not possible to give an assessment of the treatment as they did not know the indication for prescriptions and do not have access to patients' medical history. Despite this, Polish pharmacists only reported an unknown location of infection in 10.8% of the dispenses. Finally, in Spain, the difference between pharmacists and other pharmacy staff was reported by multiple pharmacies. As only pharmacists are allowed to evaluate interactions and contraindications for new patients, it was suggested to exclude technicians from the study. Indeed, the registrations show a difference between pharmacists and non-pharmacists in Spain, as they checked for interactions in 44.0% and 10.5% of the dispenses, respectively, and comparably for contraindications (46.6% vs. 0%) and allergies (62.1% vs. 7.0%).

2.4. Revising the Registration Chart for the Main Study

Based on the written feedback that was provided by the participating pharmacy staff and the results obtained during registering the dispensing practice, several changes have been made to the registration chart (Appendix B). Firstly, the total number of answer options was reduced from 46 to 39. This was achieved by changing the location of infection from a choice of infections to a known/unknown question and by removing the domain of delayed prescribing, as this occurred in less than 1% of the dispenses. Metronidazole was added to the domain of antibiotics on request of several pharmacists. Within the domain of advice, some specifications and changes were made. General advice of taking antibiotics with or without food/drinks was changed to more specifically alcohol and dairy products. The advice "do not take shortly before sleeping" and "advice regarding comedication" has been removed from the chart, as the first one was crossed in less than 1% of the dispenses, and for the latter, it is not possible to judge whether this is appropriate due to lack of information of other drug use.

3. Discussion

Antibiotic dispensing in community pharmacies is complex and varying practices within countries and across borders exist. This study shows that a simple tool to measure the antibiotic dispensing process can be implemented in community pharmacy practice. When it comes to antibiotic dispensing in community pharmacies, practice does not seem to match EU guidelines. On the one hand, this could mean that proper guidelines should be based on a real-life setting involving practicing pharmacists in establishing such guidelines. On the other hand, registration of dispensing practices using the APO methodology reveals many possibilities for improvement, although the emphasis of such improvements should be dependent on contextual factors within and between countries.

3.1. Strengths of the Study

This is the first testing of the APO methodology in community pharmacy practice. The APO methodology has been proven to be effective in general practice over several decades [7,8,10]. During this study, there was close collaboration with the initial developers of the APO methodology in general practice. In addition, the study was conducted in multiple pharmacies in countries with different antibiotic usage and community pharmacy practices. The developed registration chart was easily implemented in all these contexts, suggesting similar high feasibility in a wider range of countries, especially in the EU. Moreover, feedback from the twenty participating pharmacies has been thoroughly reviewed and led to considerable changes to the content of the registration chart, thus improving the adaptation to the field of daily practice. Finally, the research group consisted of a wide range of experts, including experts of the 5 target countries, and practicing community pharmacists.

3.2. Limitations of the Study

The complexity of the dispensing process makes it difficult to measure all topics related to it on a registration chart that can be completed within a few minutes. Within that framework, we attempted to include the most relevant parts of the antibiotic dispensing process but had to eliminate or simplify many topics from the registration chart. Several topics have been discussed and considered but not included in the final registration chart.

These include registration of multiple other antibiotics and antibiotic classes, symptom assessment of patients without an antibiotic prescription, the patients' perspective on the dispensing process, patient's adherence to antibiotic therapy, the use of point-of-care tests, the use of "wait-and-see" prescriptions, and more specific details on safety checks and a wider range of possible appropriate advice. Through this method we developed a registration chart that takes little time to complete. Nevertheless, completing the chart during dispensing will take up additional time of pharmacists, which may mean that implementation might not be possible in all pharmacies for all antibiotic dispenses.

Although it was estimated that the use of antibiotics without a prescription comprised about 7% of total antibiotic use in the EU [11], over-the-counter supply of antibiotics has not been taken up in this pilot study because the extent to which over-the-counter supply occurs differs between the four countries. Moreover, as over-the-counter supply of antibiotics is illegal in the EU, data obtained on this through a self-registry chart might not have been accurate. Other limitations include the limited number of recruited pharmacies in France and the voluntary and non-random participation of participants in the other countries. This does probably mean that the participating pharmacists are more aware of their dispensing practices, they are among the more guideline compliant pharmacists and therefore the results could be biased towards better dispensing practices than what actually happens during daily practice. Moreover, the registration chart was kept consistent for the five target countries, even though pharmacy practice differs between them. This could mean that certain topics on the registration chart may be more relevant in certain countries compared to others. Nevertheless, the final version of the registration chart was developed based on feedback from all countries, where especially those topics that seemed relevant in all contexts were included. Finally, no demographic data were collected for the participating pharmacies, e.g., related to location and size of the pharmacies.

3.3. Comparison with Literature

There is only limited literature available on documenting dispensing practice, even more so for antibiotics specifically. Cerqueira Santos et al. [6] reviewed all documentation of dispensing, but included studies mainly focusing on drug-related problems, patient information, and clinical interventions. Although such information seems to be essential for improving pharmacy services, it does not provide information on what exactly happens during the dispensing process. As dispensing practice should differ for different drug classes, specified documentation methods are needed for specific drug classes to ensure obtaining detailed information, which can be used for specific improvements in practice. Studies that focus on antibiotic dispensing have been performed around the globe [12–21], but mainly aim to identify patterns in dispensing practices, e.g., regarding the type of antibiotic dispensed or over-the-counter dispensing of antibiotics. Such studies seem very relevant to picture general antibiotic use; nonetheless, they might not be as useful in providing specific improvements for community pharmacy practice. As the methodology of this study deviates from earlier research, i.e., the APO methodology has never been used in community pharmacies before, a straightforward comparison with previous literature is difficult to make. Nevertheless, based on the feedback received from the participating pharmacists, it seems that developing and implementing an antibiotic dispensing documentation tool has been feasible and successful. Differences in community pharmacy practice throughout Europe have been reported earlier [22]. Also, with specific regard to the differences in antibiotic use and dispensing practices throughout Europe as shown in this study, similar findings have been published [23] and varied reasons have been identified, including lack of public knowledge and awareness, access to antibiotics without prescription and leftover antibiotics, knowledge and perception of prescribers and dispensers and many others [11,16,24–27]. However, care must be taken interpreting the data of this pilot study, a study on a larger scale is needed to confirm these.

3.4. Meaning of the Study and Future Studies

The ECDC has described a large role for the community pharmacist towards improving the quality of antibiotic use and therewith reducing antimicrobial resistance [3]. Nonetheless, there seems to be a large gap between the role as defined in theory and how community pharmacists fulfil this role in practice. This shows through the few safety checks that are performed and little advice that is given during dispensing and the minimal contact between pharmacists and prescribers. To diminish this gap, strengthen the role of the pharmacist in antibiotic use and hence improve antibiotic dispensing practices, it is essential that two conditions are met. Firstly, a clear picture of current practice is needed to identify problems and possibilities for improvement. The tool we developed in this pilot study might be one method to achieve this, although implementation on a larger scale would provide more convincing evidence. Secondly, pharmacists must be made aware of their role as a gatekeeper as described in the aforementioned guidelines and be given support to change their practice accordingly. It will be important that pharmacists take an active role in this change, looking for multidisciplinary collaboration (e.g., with prescribers) where possible, and striving to improve their practice from within their own profession. Part of the main study of the HAPPY PATIENT project will therefore aim to let community pharmacists gain insight in their daily practice and improve their practice according to EU guidelines using the successfully tested APO methodology [28].

4. Materials and Methods

4.1. Study Design

This pilot study is part of the Health Alliance for Prudent Prescription and Yield of Antibiotics in a Patient-centered Perspective (HAPPY PATIENT) project. This project aims to further implement the EU AMR guidelines on the prudent use of antimicrobials in humans [3]. The project is supported by the EU Third Health Programme (ID 900024) and focusses on four settings: community pharmacies, general practice, out-of-hour services, and nursing homes. The study protocol has recently been published [28].

4.2. Study Setting

Data collection was attempted in 25 community pharmacies, five pharmacies in five different countries with differences in scale and patterns of antibiotic use [29], and spread over different parts of the European Union: France, Greece, Lithuania, Poland, and Spain. Due to difficulties with pharmacist recruitment, only two pharmacists participated in France. To protect the privacy of the French participants, these results were not included in this paper. The local partners in the four countries recruited pharmacists and/or pharmacist technicians working in community pharmacies. Participating staff did not need to speak English as all materials were forward-backward translated into local languages by the local partners. There were no limitations based on pharmacy size, location, or other factors for inclusion in the study.

4.3. Development of the Registration Chart

The layout of the registration chart, with multiple variables categorized within overarching domains, was kept consistent with the original audit chart developed for GP practice as earlier published [9,10]. The content of the registration chart was adjusted to suit community pharmacy practice in the target countries. A first draft of the registration chart was developed by ML based on information from two documents: (1) a context analysis of community pharmacy practice in the target countries using a questionnaire which was completed by the local partners of the HAPPY PATIENT project; and (2) the EU AMR guidelines on the prudent use of antimicrobial for humans [3]. Further development of the registration chart, with specification of its domains and variables, was done through online discussion and consensus meetings. The core research group, M.L., R.B., and K.T., determined the focus of the registration chart by selecting appropriate domains and variables, in light of WHO [30,31] and ECDC [3] reports and the official Summary of Product Characteristics (SmPC) texts for antibiotics. For all antibiotics or antibiotic classes included in the registration chart, the SmPC texts were searched for information on recommendations and warnings for use, contraindications, interactions, and precautions. To illustrate, SmPC texts warn for photosensitivity when using tetracyclines, therefore pharmacists are expected to inform patients to be careful with sun- and UV-light when dispensing tetracyclines. Consequently, this advice was included in the registration chart.

The registration chart has been discussed during several meetings with expert groups: the developers of the original GP registration chart, local partners in the target countries, practicing community pharmacists and the complete HAPPY PATIENT project group. The list of antibiotics and antibiotic classes included in the registration chart was composed in collaboration with the local and clinical partners, for consistency throughout the project. The registration chart comprised nine domains with a total of 46 variables related to antibiotic dispensing, and two patient variables—age and sex (Appendix C); it focused on oral antibiotic prescriptions that are dispensed in the community pharmacy. The same chart was used in all four countries.

4.4. Data Collection

The registration chart and an instruction document (Appendix D) were distributed among the staff of the participating pharmacies. The instruction document provided general information about the duration of the pilot study, the in- and exclusion criteria for registering, and specific information on the nine domains of the registration chart. Specifically, pharmacy staff was instructed to register all oral antibiotic dispensing inside the pharmacy during 5 working days in October 2021. Antibiotics dispensed outside the pharmacy, e.g., deliveries to patients, were excluded. Any antibiotics prescribed for prophylactic or veterinary use were also excluded from the study. The registration charts were completed on paper, immediately after dispensing. Additionally, a list of antibiotics was provided to support pharmacy staff in assigning specific antibiotics to the appropriate antibiotic class on the registration chart. This list comprised general antibiotics for all countries (Appendix E) and was complemented with country-specific antibiotics and brand names by the local partners in the target countries. Pharmacy staff was instructed to return the charts by postal courier or digital scans to the partners in the target countries. All data were transcribed to IBM® SPSS® and Stata™ files by partners at the Research Unit for General Practice, Institute of Public Health of the University of Southern Denmark.

4.5. Questionnaire

To assess the feasibility of implementing the registration chart in practice and to acquire feedback on the registration chart, the pharmacy's staff was requested to complete a questionnaire following the pilot study (Appendix E). This questionnaire comprised ten questions, on ease of use of the documents (registration chart, instruction form, list of antibiotics), time needed for registrations, possibility to register all antibiotics in the study period, appropriateness of domains and variables, and willingness to participate among the members of the pharmacy's staff.

4.6. Data Analysis

All answers to the questionnaire were translated to English by the partners in the target countries. Due to the small number of participating pharmacies, the received feedback was discussed by the core research group in full. Any unclarities were solved, and suggestions towards increasing the ease of use of the documents or reducing the time needed to complete them were considered if these were relevant in all target countries. Similarly, the content of the registration chart was adjusted based on this questionnaire. To this extent, any topic suggested to include or remove was discussed within the core research group and compared to WHO and ECDC reports and SmPC texts. Topics mentioned by multiple pharmacists were given a higher priority. Any topic was only included if deemed relevant in all four countries and consistent with EU AMR guidelines. Additionally, the data collected with the registration chart was used to further improve its contents.

The data collected with the registration chart were also used to illustrate community pharmacy practice regarding antibiotic dispensing using Stata/MP 16. Data were analyzed descriptively for pharmacies per country and for the countries together. Crosstabs of different combinations of domains were created to analyze combinations of dispensed antibiotics and provided advice. Appropriateness of advice was determined by comparing the collected data to SmPC information for the specific antibiotics. Safety checks of contraindications, interactions, and allergies were deemed to have to be performed for all dispensed antibiotics, as described as the role of the pharmacists in the EU AMR guidelines [3].

5. Conclusions

The registration chart based on the APO methodology appears to be a feasible way to obtain detailed data on the antibiotic dispensing practices in community pharmacies. Pharmacists from different countries have been able to implement the registration chart in their daily practice. Although the complex process of antibiotic dispensing cannot be documented entirely within a few minutes, this tool does make it possible to obtain useful information about antibiotic dispensing. Nevertheless, the effectiveness of this tool is not solely based on its design; it will substantially depend on the implementation of interventions that result from using the tool in practice. This pilot study indicates the presence of considerable inconsistencies between the EU guidelines on dispensing and the everyday practices in the pharmacies.

Author Contributions: Conceptualization, M.L., R.B., J.L., M.P.H., C.L. and K.T.; methodology, M.L., R.B., J.L., M.P.H. and K.T.; formal analysis, M.L., R.B. and K.T.; investigation, M.L., R.B., A.C., C.L., P.T., I.T., M.-N.K., A.K. and K.T.; resources, M.L., R.B., A.C., J.L., M.P.H., C.L., P.T., I.T., M.-N.K., A.K. and K.T.; data curation, A.C., J.L., M.P.H., C.L., P.T., I.T., M.-N.K. and A.K.; writing—original draft preparation, M.L.; writing—review and editing, R.B., A.C., J.L., M.P.H., C.L., P.T., I.T., M.-N.K., A.K. and K.T.; supervision, K.T.; project administration, M.L.; funding acquisition, C.L. All authors have read and agreed to the published version of the manuscript.

Funding: This publication was funded by the European Union's Third Health Programme (2014–2020), project ID 900024. In Poland, this publication was also part of an international project co-financed by the program of the Ministry of Science and Higher Education entitled "PMW" in the years 2022–2023; contract no. 5241/HP3/2022/2. The funding organizations had no role in study design or concept or approval of manuscript.

Institutional Review Board Statement: Not applicable.

Informed Consent Statement: Informed consent was obtained from all subjects involved in the study.

Data Availability Statement: The data presented in this study are available on request from the corresponding author. The data are not publicly available due to the small number of participating pharmacists and their privacy.

Acknowledgments: The authors would like to thank all partners of the HAPPY PATIENT consortium for their contribution to this research, with specific thanks to all partners in the target countries who have recruited and collected the data and to the partners at the Research Unit for General Practice, Institute of public health of the University of Southern Denmark for their help with the processing of the data. Additionally, the authors thank Liset van Dijk for critically reviewing the manuscript.

Conflicts of Interest: C.L. reports grants from Abbott Diagnostics not related to this study. All other authors declare no competing interests. The funders had no role in the design of the study; in the collection, analyses, or interpretation of data; in the writing of the manuscript; or in the decision to publish the results.

Appendix A Additional Data

Table A1. Treatment duration in days of the prescribed antibiotics and advice provided during dispensing for the four countries together.

Treatment Duration in Days	Total	Total (%)	Missing 7 (1.7%)
1	5	1.2	
2	26	6.4	
3	30	7.3	
4	3	0.7	
5	42	10.3	
6	21	5.1	
7	131	32.0	
8	15	3.7	
9	5	1.2	
10	59	14.4	
11	1	0.2	
12	4	1.0	
13	1	0.2	
14	7	1.7	
15	2	0.5	
16	1	0.2	
20	9	2.2	
21	1	0.2	
30	3	0.7	
42	1	0.2	
44	1	0.2	
90	1	0.2	
98	3	0.7	
unknown	28	6.9	
Advice provided			
Treatment duration	271	66.3	
Risk of AMR	74	18.1	
Take shortly before sleeping	17	4.2	
Do not take shortly before sleeping	3	0.7	
Take with food or drinks	45	11.0	
Do not take with food or drinks	44	10.8	
Take while sitting or standing	0	0.0	
Advice regarding comedication	35	8.6	
Be careful with sunlight	20	4.9	
Information about side effects	85	20.8	
Seek medical help if symptoms worsen	76	18.6	
Bring back leftovers	15	3.7	
No advice given	52	12.7	

Table A2. Pharmacist judgement of prescription and access to prescription information (indication of infection and treatment duration (TRD).

	Indication Known		Indication Unknown	
	TRD Known	TRD Unknown	TRD Known	TRD Unknown
Agree	0	5	26	0
Insufficient info	0	14	10	9

Appendix B

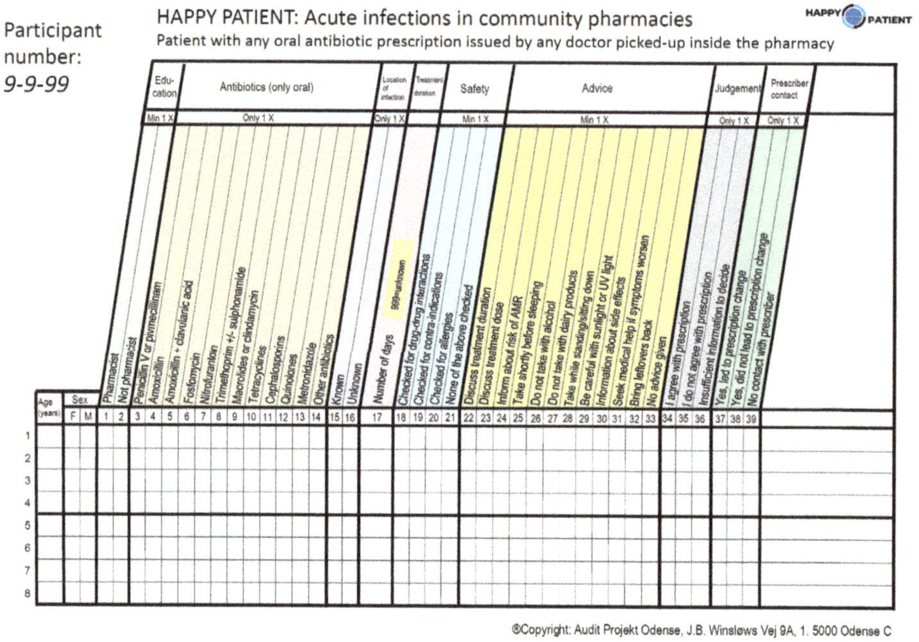

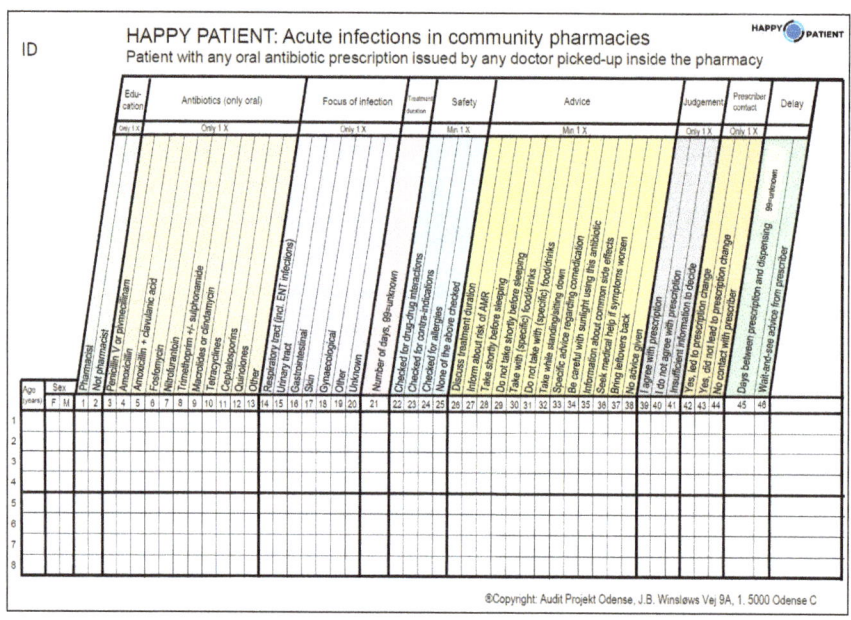

Figure A1. Final registration chart.

Appendix C

Figure A2. APO registration chart used for the pilot study. ENT: Ear, Nose and Throat.

Appendix D Instructions for Completing the APO Registration Chart

Please register for 5 days during dispensing of any oral antibiotic course. Please fill in one line for each time you dispense the antibiotic. If a patient receives multiple antibiotics, please fill in different lines for each antibiotic. We recommend using a new registration chart every day and that the registration is performed immediately after the consultation. Please find below the instructions to fill in the registration chart.

Age	Please provide age in years. For children ages less than one year, please indicate 0.
Sex	Please state if the patient is female or male.
Occupation	Please indicate if the person who has dispensed the antibiotic is a pharmacist or another staff member of the pharmacy (e.g., pharmacist technician).
Antibiotics (only oral)	Please cross (X) which antibiotic (class) has been dispensed. If necessary, please use the list provided to determine the antibiotic class to which the prescribed antibiotic belongs.
Focus infection	Please cross for which type of infection the antibiotic was prescribed. Cross unknown if this information was not available.
Treatment duration	Please state the duration of the prescribed treatment in numbers. Use 99 if the treatment length was not specified on the prescription.
Safety (multiple answers possible)	Please indicate which checks have been performed during dispensing. Drug-drug interactions include interactions with all other medication used by the patient. Contra-indications may include all conditions, states, or diseases of a patient. Allergies include all allergies to the prescribed antibiotic and any cross-reactivity reactions related to them. Multiple answers may be crossed.
Advice (multiple answers possible)	Please cross the boxes that state the advice you provided to the patient during dispensing. Multiple answers may be crossed.
Agree with the prescription	Please indicate if you agree with the prescribed antibiotic in this specific situation. Please only include disagreements on a clinical basis (e.g., antibiotic unnecessary, wrong choice of antibiotic, wrong dose/duration). Disagreement with the prescription due to administrative reasons (missing patient/prescriber information) should not be included.
Prescriber contact	Please state if contact between you and the prescriber has led to any clinical changes (e.g., change of dose/antibiotic) to the prescription. Please tick 'no contact with prescriber' if there was no additional contact between the pharmacy and the prescriber.
Delayed prescribing	Please indicate the number of days between the date of prescribing and the date of dispensing. If the antibiotic is dispensed on the same day as the prescription was issued, please indicate '0'. If this information is unknown, please indicate '99'. Please cross 'wait-and-see advice from prescriber' if the delay between prescribing and dispensing was based on advice from the prescriber. If the patients delayed on their own initiative, please leave blank.

Appendix E

Table A3. General list of antibiotics to be completed by local partners.

	Generic Name	Class
1.	Amoxicillin	Amoxicillin
2.	Amoxicillin and beta-lactamase inhibitor	Amoxicillin + clavulanic acid
3.	Azithromycin	Macrolides or clindamycin
4.	Cefadroxil	Cephalosporins
5.	Cefprozil	Cephalosporins
6.	Cefuroxime	Cephalosporins
7.	Ciprofloxacin	Quinolones
8.	Clarithromycin	Macrolides or clindamycin
9.	Clindamycin	Macrolides or clindamycin
10.	Doxycycline	Tetracyclines
11.	Erythromycin	Macrolides or clindamycin
12.	Fosfomycin	Fosfomycin
13.	Levofloxacin	Quinolones
14.	Nitrofurantoin	Nitrofurantoin
15.	Phenoxymethylpenicillin	Penicillin V or pivmecillinam
16.	Pivmecillinam	Penicillin V or pivmecillinam
17.	Sulfamethoxazole and trimethoprim	Trimethoprim +/− sulfonamide
18.	Tetracycline	Tetracyclines
19.	Trimethoprim	Trimethoprim +/− sulfonamide

Appendix F Questionnaire to Provide Feedback after Pilot Study

(1) Are the instruction document and registration chart clear/easy to use? Please specify any possible improvements.
(2) Was it easy to match the dispensed products with the antibiotic classes using the list of antibiotics provided? If not, please specify the problems you encountered.
(3) Please state how much time it takes to fill in one registration chart.
(4) Did you manage to register all patients with a prescription for an oral antibiotic for days? If not, please specify the problems you encountered.
(5) Do you believe it to be possible to register all antibiotic dispensing for a period of four weeks?
(6) Has the complete pharmacy staff participated in the pilot study or only a part of the staff?
(7) Does the advice seem appropriate to the pharmacy setting in your country?
(8) Are there any important topics/advises missing in the registration chart?
(9) Are there any topics/advises you would consider irrelevant?
(10) Do you have any additional comments?

References

1. Rusic, D.; Bozic, J.; Bukic, J.; Vilovic, M.; Tomicic, M.; Seselja Perisin, A.; Leskur, D.; Modun, D.; Cohadzic, T.; Tomic, S. Antimicrobial Resistance: Physicians' and Pharmacists' Perspective. *Microb. Drug Resist.* **2020**, *27*, 670–677. [CrossRef] [PubMed]
2. Rusic, D.; Bukić, J.; Perisin, A.S.; Leskur, D.; Modun, D.; Petric, A.; Vilovic, M.; Bozic, J. Are We Making the Most of Community Pharmacies? Implementation of Antimicrobial Stewardship Measures in Community Pharmacies: A Narrative Review. *Antibiotics* **2021**, *10*, 63. [CrossRef] [PubMed]
3. European Centre for Disease Prevention and Control *EU Guidelines for the Prudent Use of Antimicrobials in Human Health*; ECDC: Stockholm, Sweden, 2017.

4. World Health Organization. *International Pharmaceutical Federation Joint FIP/WHO Guidelines on Good Pharmacy Practice: Standards for Quality of Pharmacy Services Background*; World Health Organization: Geneva, Switzerland, 2011.
5. World Health Organization Regional Office for Europe. *The Legal and Regulatory Framework for Community Pharmacies in the WHO European Region*; World Health Organization Regional Office for Europe: Copenhagen, Denmark, 2019.
6. Santos, S.C.; Boaventura, T.C.; Rocha, K.S.S.; Filho, A.D.D.O.; Onozato, T.; de Lyra, D.P., Jr. Can we document the practice of dispensing? A systematic review. *J. Clin. Pharm. Ther.* **2016**, *41*, 634–644. [CrossRef] [PubMed]
7. Munck, A.; Damsgaard, J.; Gp, M.D.; Gilsa, D.; Hansen, Ê.; Bjerrum, L.; Sùndergaard, J. The Nordic Method for Quality Improvement in General Practice. *Qual. Prim. Care* **2003**, *11*, 73–78.
8. Llor, C.; Cots, J.M.; Hernández, S.; Ortega, J.; Arranz, J.; Monedero, M.J.; Alcántara, J.D.D.; Pérez, C.; García, G.; Gómez, M.; et al. Effectiveness of two types of intervention on antibiotic prescribing in respiratory tract infections in Primary Care in Spain. Happy Audit Study. *Atencion Primaria* **2014**, *46*, 492–500. [CrossRef]
9. Hansen, M.P.; Lykkegaard, J.; Søndergaard, J.; Munck, A.; Llor, C. How to improve practice by means of the Audit Project Odense method. *Br. J. Gen. Pract.* **2022**, *72*, 235–236. [CrossRef]
10. Munck, A.P.; Gilså Hansen, D.; Lindman, A.; Ovhed, I.; Førre, S.; Bjarni Torsteinsson, J. A Nordic Collaboration on Medical Audit: The APO method for quality development and continuous medical education (CME) in primary health care. *Scand. J. Prim. Health Care* **1998**, *16*, 2–6. [CrossRef]
11. Paget, J.; Lescure, D.; Versporten, A.; Goossens, H.; Schellevis, F.; Van Dijk, L. *Antimicrobial Resistance and Causes of Non-Prudent Use of Antibiotics in Human Medicine in the EU*; European Commission: Brussels, Belgium, 2017.
12. Torres, N.F.; Solomon, V.P.; Middleton, L.E. Pharmacists' practices for non-prescribed antibiotic dispensing in Mozambique. *Pharm. Pr.* **2020**, *18*, 1965. [CrossRef]
13. Zakaa El-din, M.; Samy, F.; Mohamed, A.; Hamdy, F.; Yasser, S.; Ehab, M. Egyptian community pharmacists' attitudes and practices towards antibiotic dispensing and antibiotic resistance; A cross-sectional survey in Greater Cairo. *Curr. Med. Res. Opin.* **2019**, *35*, 939–946. [CrossRef]
14. Darwish, R.M.; Baqain, G.N.; Aladwan, H.; Salamah, L.M.; Madi, R.; Al Masri, R.M. Knowledge, attitudes, and practices regarding antibiotic use and resistance among community pharmacists: A cross sectional study in Jordan. *Int. J. Clin. Pharm.* **2021**, *43*, 1198–1207. [CrossRef]
15. Zawahir, S.; Lekamwasam, S.; Aslani, P. Antibiotic dispensing practice in community pharmacies: A simulated client study. *Res. Soc. Adm. Pharm.* **2018**, *15*, 584–590. [CrossRef] [PubMed]
16. Zapata-Cachafeiro, M.; Piñeiro-Lamas, M.; Guinovart, M.C.; López-Vázquez, P.M.; Vazquez-Lago, J.; Figueiras, A. Magnitude and determinants of antibiotic dispensing without prescription in Spain: A simulated patient study. *J. Antimicrob. Chemother.* **2018**, *74*, 511–514. [CrossRef] [PubMed]
17. Bianco, A.; Licata, F.; Trovato, A.; Napolitano, F.; Pavia, M. Antibiotic-Dispensing Practice in Community Pharmacies: Results of a Cross-Sectional Study in Italy. *Antimicrob. Agents Chemother.* **2021**, *65*, e02729-20. [CrossRef] [PubMed]
18. Plachouras, D.; Kavatha, D.; Antoniadou, A.; Giannitsioti, E.; Poulakou, G.; Kanellakopoulou, K.; Giamarellou, H. Dispensing of antibiotics without prescription in Greece, 2008: Another link in the antibiotic resistance chain. *Eurosurveillance* **2010**, *15*, 19488. [CrossRef] [PubMed]
19. Islam, A.; Akhtar, Z.; Hassan, Z.; Chowdhury, S.; Rashid, M.; Aleem, M.A.; Ghosh, P.K.; Mah-E-Muneer, S.; Parveen, S.; Ahmmed, K.; et al. Pattern of Antibiotic Dispensing at Pharmacies According to the WHO Access, Watch, Reserve (AWaRe) Classification in Bangladesh. *Antibiotics* **2022**, *11*, 247. [CrossRef] [PubMed]
20. Nguyen, T.T.P.; Do, T.X.; Nguyen, H.A.; Nguyen, C.T.T.; Meyer, J.C.; Godman, B.; Skosana, P.; Nguyen, B.T. A National Survey of Dispensing Practice and Customer Knowledge on Antibiotic Use in Vietnam and the Implications. *Antibiotics* **2022**, *11*, 1091. [CrossRef]
21. Ndaki, P.M.; Mushi, M.F.; Mwanga, J.R.; Konje, E.T.; Ntinginya, N.E.; Mmbaga, B.T.; Keenan, K.; Sabiiti, W.; Kesby, M.; Benitez-Paez, F.; et al. Dispensing Antibiotics without Prescription at Community Pharmacies and Accredited Drug Dispensing Outlets in Tanzania: A Cross-Sectional Study. *Antibiotics* **2021**, *10*, 1025. [CrossRef]
22. *Institute for Evidence-Based Health Pharmacy Services in Europe: Evaluating Trends and Value*; ISBE: Lisbon, Portugal, 2020.
23. Kaae, S.; Ghazaryan, L.; Pagava, K.; Korinteli, I.; Makalkina, L.; Zhetimkarinova, G.; Ikhambayeva, A.; Tentiuc, E.; Ratchina, S.; Zakharenkova, P.; et al. The antibiotic knowledge, attitudes and behaviors of patients, doctors and pharmacists in the WHO Eastern European region—A qualitative, comparative analysis of the culture of antibiotic use in Armenia, Georgia, Kazakhstan, Moldova, Russia and Tajikistan. *Res. Soc. Adm. Pharm.* **2020**, *16*, 238–248. [CrossRef]
24. Machowska, A.; Lundborg, C.S. Drivers of Irrational Use of Antibiotics in Europe. *Int. J. Environ. Res. Public Health* **2019**, *16*, 27. [CrossRef]
25. Servia-Dopazo, M.; Figueiras, A. Determinants of antibiotic dispensing without prescription: A systematic review. *J. Antimicrob. Chemother.* **2018**, *73*, 3244–3253. [CrossRef]
26. Roque, F.; Soares, S.; Breitenfeld, L.; López-Durán, A.; Figueiras, A.; Herdeiro, M.T. Attitudes of community pharmacists to antibiotic dispensing and microbial resistance: A qualitative study in Portugal. *Int. J. Clin. Pharm.* **2013**, *35*, 417–424. [CrossRef] [PubMed]
27. Lescure, D.; Paget, J.; Schellevis, F.; Van Dijk, L. Determinants of Self-Medication with Antibiotics in European and Anglo-Saxon Countries: A Systematic Review of the Literature. *Front. Public Health* **2018**, *6*, 370. [CrossRef] [PubMed]

28. Bjerrum, A.; García-Sangenís, A.; Modena, D.; Córdoba, G.; Bjerrum, L.; Chalkidou, A.; Lykkegaard, J.; Hansen, M.P.; Søndergaard, J.; Nexøe, J.; et al. Health alliance for prudent prescribing and yield of antibiotics in a patient-centred perspective (HAPPY PATIENT): A before-and-after intervention and implementation study protocol. *BMC Prim. Care* **2022**, *23*, 102. [CrossRef] [PubMed]
29. *European Centre for Disease Prevention and Control Summary of the Latest Data on Antibiotic Consumption in the European Union*; ECDC: Stockholm, Sweden, 2017.
30. World Health Organization Regional Office for Europe. *European Strategic Action Plan on Antibiotic Resistance*; World Health Organization Regional Office for Europe: Copenhagen, Denmark, 2011.
31. World Health Organization Regional Office for Europe. *The Role of Pharmacist in Encouraging Prudent Use of Antibiotics and Averting Antimicrobial Resistance: A Review of Policy and Experience*; World Health Organization Regional Office for Europe: Copenhagen, Denmark, 2014.

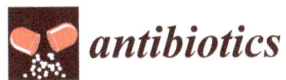

Brief Report

The Effect of the COVID-19 Pandemic on Outpatient Antibiotic Prescription Rates in Children and Adolescents—A Claims-Based Study in Germany

Manas K. Akmatov [1,*], Claudia Kohring [1], Lotte Dammertz [1], Joachim Heuer [1], Maike Below [2], Jörg Bätzing [1] and Jakob Holstiege [1]

1. Department of Epidemiology and Health Care Atlas, Central Research Institute of Ambulatory Health Care, 10587 Berlin, Germany
2. Department of Prescription Data, Central Research Institute of Ambulatory Health Care, 10587 Berlin, Germany
* Correspondence: makmatov@zi.de; Tel.: +49-(0)30-4005-2414

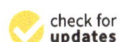

Citation: Akmatov, M.K.; Kohring, C.; Dammertz, L.; Heuer, J.; Below, M.; Bätzing, J.; Holstiege, J. The Effect of the COVID-19 Pandemic on Outpatient Antibiotic Prescription Rates in Children and Adolescents—A Claims-Based Study in Germany. *Antibiotics* 2022, 11, 1433. https://doi.org/10.3390/antibiotics11101433

Academic Editors: Ria Benkő and Gyöngyvér Soós

Received: 30 September 2022
Accepted: 17 October 2022
Published: 18 October 2022

Publisher's Note: MDPI stays neutral with regard to jurisdictional claims in published maps and institutional affiliations.

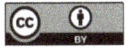

Copyright: © 2022 by the authors. Licensee MDPI, Basel, Switzerland. This article is an open access article distributed under the terms and conditions of the Creative Commons Attribution (CC BY) license (https://creativecommons.org/licenses/by/4.0/).

Abstract: The aim of the study was to examine whether the COVID-19 pandemic had any effect on antibiotic prescription rates in children in Germany. Using the nationwide outpatient prescription data from the Statutory Health Insurance from 2010 to 2021, changes in the monthly prescriptions of systemic antibiotics dispensed to children aged 0–14 years were examined (n = 9,688,483 in 2021). Interrupted time series analysis was used to assess the effect of mitigation measures against SARS-COV-2, introduced in March and November 2020, on antibiotic prescription rates. In the pre-pandemic period, the antibiotic prescription rates displayed a linear decrease from 2010 to 2019 (mean annual decrease, −6%). In 2020, an immediate effect of mitigation measures on prescription rates was observed; in particular, the rate decreased steeply in April (RR 0.24, 95% CI: 0.14–0.41) and November 2020 (0.44, 0.27–0.73). The decrease was observed in all ages and for all antibiotic subgroups. However, this effect was temporary. Regionally, prescription rates were highly correlated between 2019 and 2020/2021. Substantial reductions in antibiotic prescription rates following the mitigation measures may indicate limited access to medical care, changes in care-seeking behavior and/or a decrease of respiratory infections. Despite an all-time low of antibiotic use, regional variations remained high and strongly correlated with pre-pandemic levels.

Keywords: adolescents; antibiotics; children; COVID-19; claims data; Germany; prescription rates; SARS-CoV-2

1. Introduction

An increasing number of studies has shown that the COVID-19 pandemic and associated public health measures affected the epidemiology of other infectious diseases. As compared to the pre-pandemic period, the incidence of both viral and bacterial infections decreased. For example, the Robert Koch Institute in Germany reported the decrease in the number of notifiable cases for all infectious diseases, except tick-borne encephalitis [1,2]. In addition, several countries, including Australia [3], England [4], Scotland [5], Canada [6] and the USA [7], observed the reduction in antibiotic prescriptions in the early phase of the pandemic. A similar trend has been observed in Europe; surveillance data showed a reduction of antibiotic use in the general population in outpatient and hospital prescriptions combined between 2019 and 2020 of 17.6% [8]. Prior to the COVID-19 pandemic, the antibiotic prescription rate in children and adolescents had been decreasing constantly since 2010 in Germany [9,10]. Namely, the antibiotic prescription rate decreased significantly from 746 prescriptions per 1000 children in 2010 to 428 per 1000 in 2018. In the current study, we examined whether there was a similar association of the COVID-19 pandemic and associated mitigation measures against SARS-CoV-2 with the prescription of antibiotics in Germany compared to the above-mentioned countries. The first mitigation measures against SARS-CoV-2 were introduced in March 2020 and lasted two months (so-called lockdown). They comprised the closure of day-care centers, schools, leisure amenities and extensive contact restrictions (up to two persons). On 2 November 2020, a second set of mitigation measures (so-called lockdown light) was implemented and included contact reduction (up to 10 persons from the same household etc.). However, as the COVID-19 case numbers continued to rise, on 15 December 2020, the mitigation measures were extended until May 2021.

2. Results

In the pre-pandemic period between 2010 and 2019, the prescription rates displayed an expected seasonal pattern, with the highest prescription rates in December, January and February and the lowest rates in July. Overall, the secular trend was decreasing from 749 per 1000 children in 2010 to 401 per 1000 children in 2019, with a mean annual decrease of 6% (Figure 1a and Table 1). In 2020 and 2021, we observed a more pronounced decline (−43% and −53% compared to 2019). In particular, the prescription rate started decreasing steeply in April 2020 (9 prescriptions per 1000 children compared to 35 prescriptions in March 2020) (Figure 1a). We observed an immediate significant effect of both the first and second lockdowns on antibiotic prescription rates (Table 1). The decrease following the first lockdown was stronger (RR, 0.24; 95% CI: 0.14–0.41) than after the second lockdown (RR, 0.44, 95% CI: 0.27–0.73). The decrease in prescription rates during the COVID-19 pandemic was observed in all ages (Figure 1b,c) and for all antibiotic subgroups (Figure 2 and Table S3). However, the effect of both lockdowns was temporary; in the months after the end of the mitigation measures, prescription rates increased (Figure 1a and Table 1). This increase in 2021, however, was age-dependent and more pronounced in children aged five years and under, and less pronounced in children and adolescents aged 6–18 years (Figure 1b,c).

In 2019, the year before the COVID-19 pandemic, the antibiotic prescription rates varied regionally by a factor of 1.9 from 294 prescriptions in Brandenburg (East Germany) to 566 prescriptions per 1000 children in Saarland (West Germany). Antibiotic prescriptions in 2019 correlated strongly with those from 2020 (Spearman's rho = 0.95, $p < 0.0001$, Figure 3) and 2021 (rho = 0.84, $p < 0.0001$).

Table 1. Effect of mitigation measures against SARS-Cov-2 on monthly antibiotic prescription rates in children in Germany—results of a generalized linear model with a Poisson distribution, 2010 to 2021.

Variables	Coefficient	Adjusted RR *	95% CI	p Value
Time since the study start (months)	−0.005	0.995	0.994–0.995	**<0.0001**
First lockdown				
Yes	**−1.422**	**0.24**	**0.14–0.41**	**<0.0001**
No		ref.		
Post-first-lockdown period (months)	0.097	1.10	0.98–1.23	0.087
Second lockdown				
Yes	**−0.812**	**0.44**	**0.27–0.73**	**0.002**
No		ref.		
Post-second-lockdown period (months)	0.009	1.01	0.90–1.13	0.873

* Adjusted for all variables in the table. Statistically significant findings are in bold. RR, relative risk; CI, confidence intervals.

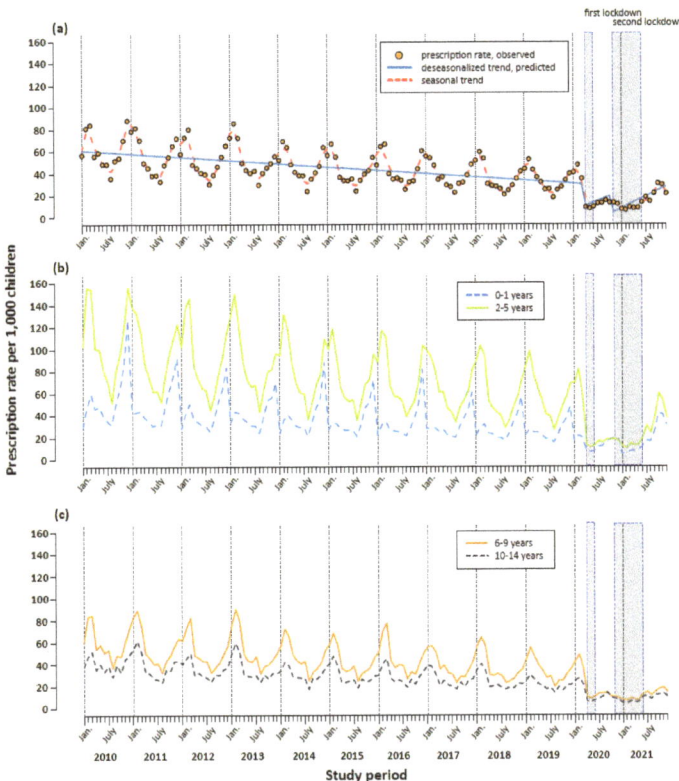

Figure 1. Trends in monthly antibiotic prescription rates per 1000 children aged between 0 and 14 years (**a**) and by age group (**b**,**c**) in the period 2010 to 2021. The first lockdown was introduced on 23 March 2020 and comprised extensive contact restrictions. The second, so-called lockdown light, started on 2 November 2020. (**a**) Solid line: predicted deseasonalized trend, dashed line: seasonal trend estimated with cubic spline.

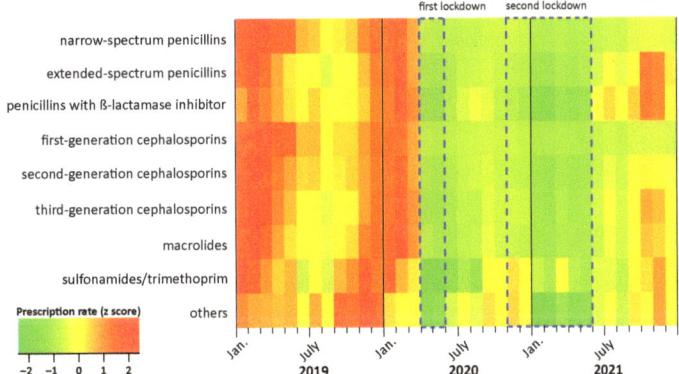

Figure 2. Trends in monthly antibiotic prescription rates per 1000 children aged between 0 and 14 years by antibiotic subgroup in the period 2019 to 2021. Original data can be found in Table S3. Values for prescription rates (x) were converted into z-scores using the formula: $x(z-score) = \frac{x - mean(x)}{SD(x)}$ to obtain mean = 0 and standard deviation (SD) = 1.

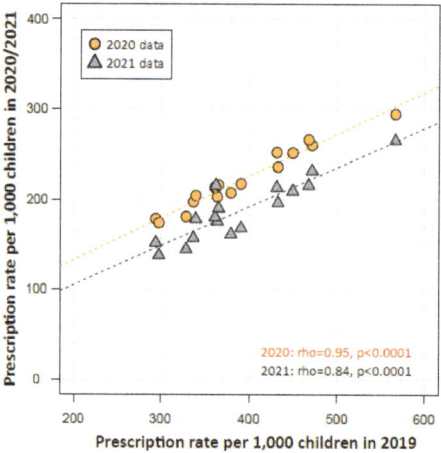

Figure 3. Scatter plot depicting the antibiotic prescription rates in regions in 2019 over its rates in 2020 and 2021. Regions are represented by the regional Associations of Statutory Health Insurance Physicians (ASHIP, $n = 17$). The Spearman's rank correlation coefficient (rho) was used to examine the relationship of the prescription rates in regional ASHIPS from the years 2019 and 2020/2021.

3. Discussion

The current study provides results from a near-real-life monitoring of outpatient antibiotic use among children and adolescents with the Statutory Health Insurance in Germany, who make up about 83% of the general population in this age segment. We observed an immediate effect of the mitigation measures against SARS-CoV-2 on total antibiotic prescription rates in all age groups, all German regions and for all antibiotic subgroups. In particular, the effect was more prominent following the first lockdown, which, among other measures, included the closure of kindergartens and schools, cancellation of leisure activities and extensive contact restrictions. Overall, the pediatric antibiotic prescription rate decreased by 43% in 2020 and by 53% in 2021 compared to its pre-pandemic level in 2019. These findings are not unexpected and have been observed in studies from other industrialized, including European, countries for the year 2020 [4,5,11]. A US study showed a decline in antibiotic dispensing in children aged 0–19 years of −27% in 2020 compared to 2019 [7]. A similar finding was observed in Canada; the total prescription rate decreased from 50 to 37 prescriptions per 1000 persons in all age groups, corresponding to a 27% reduction [6]. The strongest decline of about 70% was reported for children aged 0–18 years [6]. In contrast to these studies, we examined the simultaneous effect of risk-mitigation measures during the two pandemic years, 2020 and 2021, in Germany. This is important as both pandemic years displayed a shift from overall seasonal patterns of antibiotic use. In addition, seasonal patterns showed strong differences between both pandemic years.

The substantial reductions in prescription rates may be explained by limited access to healthcare facilities and/or changes in care-seeking behavior. However, large-scale mitigation measures against SARS-CoV-2 may also have resulted in the reduction of other infections, in particular respiratory tract infections of both viral and bacterial origin [12], up to the complete non-appearance of a typical seasonal outbreak of acute respiratory infections, such as respiratory syncytial virus in infants and toddlers or seasonal influenza in the winter season 2020/2021 [13]. Moreover, national notification data from the Robert Koch Institute observed the decrease in all other notifiable infectious diseases during the SARS-CoV-2-pandemic, with the exception of tick-borne encephalitis [1,2]. For example, about 163,000 infectious diseases (excluding SARS-CoV-2) were notified between March and July 2020. The numbers of the same notified infectious diseases were much higher before the pandemic (2016: 220,000; 2017: 196,000; 2018: 345,000; 2019: 248,000), corresponding to a relative reduction of about −35%. The highest decrease in notified infections was observed in children and adolescents (age group '0–4 years', −57% and '5–14 years', −45%) and the lowest in adults ('35–59 years', −26%). In line with the above-mentioned studies, the strongest fall was observed for respiratory tract infections, such as measles (−86%), pertussis (−64%) and *Haemophilus influenzae* (−61%). Gastrointestinal infections due to rotavirus infection (−83%) and shigellosis (−83%) also showed strong decreases.

The re-increase of antibiotic prescriptions in 2021 compared with 2019 showed age-dependency and was less pronounced in children and adolescents older than five years compared with younger children. This might be due to age-dependent variation in health-seeking behavior on the one hand. On the other hand, it cannot be excluded that the second lockdown in 2021 was implemented stricter in schools than in kindergartens. At this point in time, it is not yet possible to judge whether the stronger decline in older children and adolescents will be sustainable in the coming years.

Of note, despite an all-time low of antibiotic use, regional variations in prescription rates remained high and were strongly correlated with pre-pandemic levels. Large-scale mitigation measures against SARS-CoV-2, especially in 2020, were, for the most part, uniformly implemented in Germany and their effect on the circulation of respiratory pathogens is unlikely to have differed between German regions. Hence, the strong correlation of regional pre- and peri-pandemic prescription rates further supports the hypothesis that pre-existing antibiotic prescription paradigms are an important explanatory factor for intra-country regional variations. Future research should assess regional differences in attitudes and levels of knowledge in the community and among healthcare providers and may inform regionally tailored interventions to further promote judicious antibiotic prescribing.

Several limitations of the study are worthy of mention. Firstly, we used secondary claims data to examine the association between risk-mitigation measures and antibiotic prescribing. This is an ecological study, which cannot establish causality. Secondly, our dataset did not contain information for antibiotics dispensed (i) by outpatient dentists and (ii) inpatient prescriptions. Finally, data for children insured privately in Germany are not part of our dataset. The latter group comprise about 13% of the general population and may differ in terms of health and socio-demographic status.

4. Materials and Methods

4.1. Data and Study Population

We used nationwide outpatient prescription data from the Statutory Health Insurance (SHI) in Germany from January 2010 to December 2021 which were collected in accordance with Article 300(2) of the Social Code Book V. The data contain all prescribed and dispensed medications (excluding dental prescriptions), the date of prescription, the pharmacy dispensation date, the amount of the prescribed substance, the anatomical therapeutic chemical (ATC) code, the defined daily doses (DDD), packaging size, strength and formulation, as well as the generic and trade names. In addition, the data include information on outpatient's age in years and region of residence. The latter is represented by the regional Associations of Statutory Health Insurance Physicians (ASHIPs). In brief, there are 17 ASHIPs in Germany, 15 of them in each German federal state and two ASHIPs presenting in the federal state North-Rhine Westphalia. The study population comprised all children aged between 0 and 14 years in the respective years (n = 9,688,483 at 1 July 2021), covering approx. 83% of the total German population in this age group (Tables S1 and S2).

4.2. Antibiotics of Interest

We examined the prescription of the following systemic antibiotics: (i) penicillins with extended spectrum (J01CA), (ii) narrow-spectrum penicillins (J01CE, J01CF), (iii) Penicillins with beta-lactamase inhibitors (J01CR), (iv) first-generation cephalosporins (J01DB), (v) second-generation cephalosporins (J01DC), (vi) third-generation cephalosporins (J01DD),

(vii) sulphonamides/trimethoprim (J01EB, J01EE, and J01EA) and (viii) macrolides (J01FA). The remaining antibiotics were categorized into the group "other antibiotics".

4.3. Statistical Analysis

We calculated annual and monthly antibiotic prescription rates per 1000 children over the period 2010 to 2021, overall, as well as by age group (0–1, 2–5, 6–9 and 10–14 years), region of residence (i.e., ASHIP) and antibiotic subgroup. The total annual number of persons with SHI per age group on July 1st of a given year, derived from national statistics provided by the German Ministry of Health, was used as a denominator [14]. To examine the effect of the mitigation measures on the antibiotic prescription rate, we conducted an interrupted time series analysis using a generalized linear model with a Poisson distribution. The dependent variable was a monthly prescription rate. Since antibiotic prescribing follows a seasonal pattern, we applied seasonal decomposition to remove seasonal variation. The independent variables were: (i) time elapsed since the start of the study in months, (ii) two binary variables indicating the start of mitigation measures (i.e., first and second lockdown) and (iii) two variables for time elapsed since the introduction of each mitigation measure in months. The Spearman's rank correlation coefficient (rho) was used to examine the relationship of the prescription rates in regional ASHIPS from the years 2019 and 2020/2021. Analyses were performed with the R Foundation for Statistical Computing, version 3.3.2 (Vienna, Austria) [15].

Supplementary Materials: The following supporting information can be downloaded at: https://www.mdpi.com/article/10.3390/antibiotics11101433/s1, Table S1: The size of the total and study population in the age segment 0–14 years and annual prescription rate in Germany in the period 2010 to 2021; Table S2: The size of the total and study population in the age segment 0–14 years and annual prescription rate in 2021 by age group; Table S3: Monthly antibiotic prescription rate per 1000 children aged between 0 and 14 years by antibiotic subgroup in the period 2019 to 2021.

Author Contributions: Conceptualization, M.K.A. and J.H. (Jakob Holstiege); methodology, M.K.A. and J.H. (Jakob Holstiege); formal analysis, M.K.A. and J.H. (Jakob Holstiege); writing—original draft preparation, M.K.A. and J.H. (Jakob Holstiege); writing—review & editing, C.K., L.D., J.H. (Joachim Heuer), M.B., J.B.; visualization, M.K.A.; supervision, M.K.A. and J.H. (Jakob Holstiege). All authors have read and agreed to the published version of the manuscript.

Funding: The authors received no financial support for the research, authorship and publication of this article.

Institutional Review Board Statement: In Germany, the use of data from insurance claims for scientific research is regulated by the Social Code Book (SGB V). Ethical approval was not required as our study used routinely collected anonymized data.

Informed Consent Statement: Informed consent was not required as our study used routinely collected anonymized data.

Data Availability Statement: The datasets analyzed during the current study are not publicly available due to data protection regulations by the Social Code Book (SGB V).

Acknowledgments: The authors thank the 17 regional Associations of Statutory Health Insurance Physicians in Germany for providing the datasets.

Conflicts of Interest: The authors declare no conflict of interest.

References

1. Ullrich, A.; Schranz, M.; Rexroth, U.; Hamouda, O.; Schaade, L.; Diercke, M.; Boender, T.S.; Robert Koch's Infectious Disease Surveillance Group. Impact of the COVID-19 pandemic and associated non-pharmaceutical interventions on other notifiable infectious diseases in Germany: An analysis of national surveillance data during week 1-2. *Lancet Reg. Health Eur.* **2021**, *6*, 100103. [CrossRef] [PubMed]
2. Schranz, M.; Ulrich, A.; Hamouda, O.; Schaade, L.; Diercke, M.; Boender, S. Die Auswirkungen der COVID-19-Pandemie und assoziierter Public-Health-Maßnahmen auf andere meldepflichtige Infektionskrankheiten in Deutschland (MW 1/2016-32/2020). *Epid. Bull* **2021**, *7*, 3–7.

3. Gillies, M.B.; Burgner, D.P.; Ivancic, L.; Nassar, N.; Miller, J.E.; Sullivan, S.G.; Todd, I.M.; Pearson, S.A.; Schaffer, A.L.; Zoega, H. Changes in antibiotic prescribing following COVID-19 restrictions: Lessons for post-pandemic antibiotic stewardship. *Br. J. Clin. Pharmacol.* **2022**, *88*, 1143–1151. [CrossRef] [PubMed]
4. Andrews, A.; Budd, E.L.; Hendrick, A.; Ashiru-Oredope, D.; Beech, E.; Hopkins, S.; Gerver, S.; Muller-Pebody, B.; AMU COVID-19 Stakeholder Group. Surveillance of Antibacterial Usage during the COVID-19 Pandemic in England, 2020. *Antibiotics* **2021**, *10*, 841. [CrossRef] [PubMed]
5. Malcolm, W.; Seaton, R.A.; Haddock, G.; Baxter, L.; Thirlwell, S.; Russell, P.; Cooper, L.; Thomson, A.; Sneddon, J. Impact of the COVID-19 pandemic on community antibiotic prescribing in Scotland. *JAC Antimicrob. Resist* **2020**, *2*, dlaa105. [CrossRef] [PubMed]
6. Knight, B.D.; Shurgold, J.; Smith, G.; MacFadden, D.R.; Schwartz, K.L.; Daneman, N.; Tropper, D.G.; Brooks, J. The impact of COVID-19 on community antibiotic use in Canada: An ecological study. *Clin. Microbiol. Infect.* **2022**, *28*, 426–432. [CrossRef] [PubMed]
7. Chua, K.P.; Volerman, A.; Conti, R.M. Prescription Drug Dispensing to US Children During the COVID-19 Pandemic. *Pediatrics* **2021**, *148*, e2021049972. [CrossRef] [PubMed]
8. European Centre for Disease Prevention and Control. Antimicrobial Consumption in the EU/EEA (ESAC-Net)—Annual Epidemiological Report for 2020. ECDC. Available online: https://www.ecdc.europa.eu/en/publications-data/downloadable-tables-antimicrobial-consumption-annual-epidemiological-report-2020 (accessed on 21 September 2022).
9. Holstiege, J.; Schulz, M.; Akmatov, M.K.; Kern, W.V.; Steffen, A.; Batzing, J. The Decline in Outpatient Antibiotic Use. *Dtsch. Arztebl. Int.* **2020**, *117*, 679–686. [CrossRef] [PubMed]
10. Holstiege, J.; Schulz, M.; Akmatov, M.K.; Steffen, A.; Batzing, J. Marked reductions in outpatient antibiotic prescriptions for children and adolescents—A population-based study covering 83% of the paediatric population, Germany, 2010 to 2018. *Euro Surveill.* **2020**, *25*, 1900599. [CrossRef] [PubMed]
11. Abelenda-Alonso, G.; Padulles, A.; Rombauts, A.; Gudiol, C.; Pujol, M.; Alvarez-Pouso, C.; Jodar, R.; Carratalà, J. Antibiotic prescription during the COVID-19 pandemic: A biphasic pattern. *Infect. Control Hosp. Epidemiol.* **2020**, *41*, 1371–1372. [CrossRef] [PubMed]
12. Oh, D.Y.; Buda, S.; Biere, B.; Reiche, J.; Schlosser, F.; Duwe, S.; Wedde, M.; von Kleist, M.; Mielke, M.; Wolff, T. Trends in respiratory virus circulation following COVID-19-targeted nonpharmaceutical interventions in Germany, January–September 2020: Analysis of national surveillance data. *Lancet Reg. Health Eur.* **2021**, *6*, 100112. [CrossRef] [PubMed]
13. Lange, M.; Happle, C.; Hamel, J.; Dördelmann, M.; Bangert, M.; Kramer, R.; Eberhardt, F.; Panning, M.; Heep, A.; Hansen, G.; et al. Non-Appearance of the RSV Season 2020/21 During the COVID-19 Pandemic-Prospective, Multicenter Data on the Incidence of Respiratory Syncytial Virus (RSV) Infection. *Dtsch. Arztebl. Int.* **2021**, *118*, 561–562. [PubMed]
14. Ministry of Health. Members and Insured Persons of the Statutory Health Insurance. Statistics on Insured Persons, by Status, Age, Place of Residence and Type of Health Insurance (on 1 July of the Respective Year). Available online: https://www.bundesgesundheitsministerium.de/themen/krankenversicherung/zahlen-und-fakten-zur-krankenversicherung/mitglieder-und-versicherte.html (accessed on 1 September 2022).
15. R Core Team. *R: A Language and Environment for Statistical Computing*; Version 3.3.2.; R Foundation for Statistical Computing: Vienna, Austria, 2016; Available online: https://www.r-project.org (accessed on 5 January 2022).

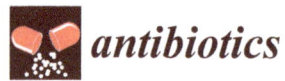

Article

Effect of Fluoroquinolone Use in Primary Care on the Development and Gradual Decay of *Escherichia coli* Resistance to Fluoroquinolones: A Matched Case-Control Study

Peter Konstantin Kurotschka [1,*], Chiara Fulgenzio [2], Roberto Da Cas [3], Giuseppe Traversa [3,4], Gianluigi Ferrante [5], Orietta Massidda [6], Ildikó Gágyor [1], Richard Aschbacher [7], Verena Moser [7], Elisabetta Pagani [7], Stefania Spila Alegiani [3] and Marco Massari [3]

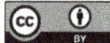

Citation: Kurotschka, P.K.; Fulgenzio, C.; Da Cas, R.; Traversa, G.; Ferrante, G.; Massidda, O.; Gágyor, I.; Aschbacher, R.; Moser, V.; Pagani, E.; et al. Effect of Fluoroquinolone Use in Primary Care on the Development and Gradual Decay of *Escherichia coli* Resistance to Fluoroquinolones: A Matched Case-Control Study. *Antibiotics* 2022, *11*, 822. https://doi.org/10.3390/antibiotics11060822

Academic Editors: Gyöngyvér Soós and Ria Benkő

Received: 31 May 2022
Accepted: 15 June 2022
Published: 18 June 2022

Publisher's Note: MDPI stays neutral with regard to jurisdictional claims in published maps and institutional affiliations.

Copyright: © 2022 by the authors. Licensee MDPI, Basel, Switzerland. This article is an open access article distributed under the terms and conditions of the Creative Commons Attribution (CC BY) license (https://creativecommons.org/licenses/by/4.0/).

[1] Department of General Practice, University Hospital Wuerzburg, Josef-Schneider-Str. 2, 97080 Wuerzburg, Germany; gagyor_i@ukw.de
[2] Pharmacy Unit, IRCCS Regina Elena National Cancer Institute and San Gallicano Institute, 00128 Rome, Italy; fulgenzio.chiara@gmail.com
[3] Pharmacoepidemiology and Pharmacovigilance Unit, National Centre for Drug Research and Evaluation, Italian National Institute of Health (ISS), 00161 Rome, Italy; roberto.dacas@iss.it (R.D.C.); g.traversa@aifa.gov.it (G.T.); stefania.spila@iss.it (S.S.A.); marco.massari@iss.it (M.M.)
[4] Italian Medicine Agency (AIFA), 00187 Rome, Italy
[5] Azienda Ospedaliera-Universitaria Città della Salute e della Scienza di Torino, 10126 Turin, Italy; gianluigi.ferrante@cpo.it
[6] Department of Cellular, Computational and Integrative Biology, Center of Medical Sciences (CISMed), University of Trento, 38122 Trento, Italy; orietta.massidda@unitn.it
[7] Health Service of the Autonomous Province of Bolzano/Bozen, 39100 Bolzano/Bozen, Italy; richard.aschbacher@sabes.it (R.A.); verena.moser@provincia.bz.it (V.M.); elisabetta.pagani@sabes.it (E.P.)
* Correspondence: kurotschka_p@ukw.de

Abstract: The reversibility of bacterial resistance to antibiotics is poorly understood. Therefore, the aim of this study was to determine, over a period of five years, the effect of fluoroquinolone (FQ) use in primary care on the development and gradual decay of *Escherichia coli* resistance to FQ. In this matched case–control study, we linked three sources of secondary data of the Health Service of the Autonomous Province of Bolzano, Italy. Cases were all those with an FQ-resistant *E. coli* (QREC)-positive culture from any site during a 2016 hospital stay. Data were analyzed using conditional logistic regression. A total of 409 cases were matched to 993 controls (FQ-sensitive *E. coli*) by the date of the first isolate. Patients taking one or more courses of FQ were at higher risk of QREC colonization/infection. The risk was highest during the first year after FQ was taken (OR 2.67, 95%CI 1.92–3.70, $p < 0.0001$), decreased during the second year (OR 1.54, 95%CI 1.09–2.17, $p = 0.015$) and became undetectable afterwards (OR 1.09, 95%CI 0.80–1.48, $p = 0.997$). In the first year, the risk of resistance was highest after greater cumulative exposure to FQs. Moreover, older age, male sex, longer hospital stays, chronic obstructive pulmonary disease (COPD) and diabetes mellitus were independent risk factors for QREC colonization/infection. A single FQ course significantly increases the risk of QREC colonization/infection for no less than two years. This risk is higher in cases of multiple courses, longer hospital stays, COPD and diabetes; in males; and in older patients. These findings may inform public campaigns and courses directed to prescribers to promote rational antibiotic use.

Keywords: drug resistance; bacterial; antimicrobial resistance; anti-bacterial agents; primary care; *Escherichia coli*; quinolones; fluoroquinolones; information storage and retrieval

1. Introduction

Antimicrobial resistance (AMR), mainly promoted by antibiotic use, is an urgent public health issue [1–3]. Its notable health and economic burdens are of global concern and have resulted in international research and policy efforts with the aim of reducing antimicrobial consumption [4,5]. One area of interest is antibiotic use in primary care, since drug resistance of pathogens causing community-acquired infections is widespread and primary care physicians are responsible for the vast majority of antibiotic prescriptions issued in the human health sector, mainly for respiratory and urinary tract infections [6,7]. Previous studies have shown a strong association between antibiotic use in primary care and the emergence of AMR, with a stronger association observed when antibiotic use is recent [8–10]. What is still poorly understood is to what extend a reversal of existing AMR may occur due to a reduction in antimicrobial use and how much time the return of antibiotic susceptibility takes in different bacterial species and after the use of specific antibiotics [8]. In a previous study conducted in the Autonomous Province of Bolzano, located in northern Italy, we found that, over a five-year period, the risk of developing a community-acquired infection due to a third-generation cephalosporin-resistant (3GC) *Escherichia coli* increases significantly in patients who were previously exposed to antibiotics. The highest risk was observed when antibiotics were taken in the last 12 months and for greater cumulative exposures to any antibiotic, as well as to 3GC [11]. Improving our knowledge of the resistance decay of different bacterial species and after exposure to different antibiotics is critical to inform antibiotic stewardship interventions and clinical decisions with the aim of minimizing AMR worldwide [12,13]. To the best of our knowledge, no study has examined the long-term effect of fluoroquinolone (FQ) use on the development and decay of FQ resistance in *E. coli* in individual patients, despite its high prevalence and the growing resistance rates, which are causing a progressive loss of efficacy of FQs in many clinical settings [14]. Therefore, we set up the present study to determine the influence of outpatient FQ use on the development and decay of FQ resistance in *E. coli*.

2. Results

Out of the 1342 patients included in the analyses, specimens derived from urine cultures accounted for 73%, followed by blood cultures, which accounted for 9%.

Within the five years of the study, 409 cases and 933 controls, with a ratio of 2.3 controls per case, were included. The sample characteristics and the results of the univariate regression analysis are shown in Table 1.

Table 1. Characteristics of case patients colonized/infected with QREC and matched control patients colonized/infected with FQ-susceptible *E. coli* and univariate conditional logistic regression analyses.

Variable	Cases [a] N = 403	Controls [a] N = 933	Crude OR (95% CI)	p
Age, Median (IQ)	78 (68–85)	74 (59–84)	1.17 [b] (1.10–1.25)	<0.0001
Gender, Male (%)	176 (43.03)	291 (31.19)	1.66 (1.30–2.11)	<0.0001
Drug's DDD taken in previous 5 years, Median (IQ)	4760 (1741–8074)	2869 (256–6190)	1.07 [c] (1.04–1.10)	<0.0001
Number of active ingredients taken in previous 5 years, Median (IQ)	17 (9–24)	10 (4–18)	1.05 (1.04–1.06)	<0.0001
At least one FQ in previous 1st year (%)	161 (39.36)	148 (15.86)	3.87 (2.88–5.18)	<0.0001
At least one FQ taken in previous 2nd year (%)	129 (31.54)	142 (15.22)	2.72 (2.04–3.64)	<0.0001
At least one FQ taken in previous 3rd, 4th or 5th year (%)	173 (42.30)	261 (27.97)	1.90 (1.49–2.44)	<0.0001
FQ prescriptions in previous year (%)				
0	248 (60.64)	785 (84.14)	Ref.	
1	72 (17.60)	83 (8.90)	3.14 (2.17–4.53)	<0.0001
2	40 (9.78)	35 (3.75)	3.80 (2.33–6.19)	<0.0001
3+	49 (11.98)	30 (3.22)	6.00 (3.55–10.17)	<0.0001
Number of hospitalizations in previous 5 years, Median (IQ)	4 (2–8)	2 (0–4)	3.67 (2.76–4.88)	<0.0001
Hospitalization days, Median (IQ)	48 (12–116)	10 (0–41)	1.07 [d] (1.05–1.09)	<0.0001

Table 1. Cont.

Variable	Cases [a] N = 403	Controls [a] N = 933	Crude OR (95% CI)	p
Hospitalization with surgery (%)	206 (50.37)	370 (39.66)	1.54 (1.23–1.95)	<0.0001
Hospitalization with device implantation (%)	44 (10.76)	65 (6.97)	1.57 (1.05–2.36)	0.029
Hospitalization with organ transplant (%)	9 (2.20)	18 (1.93)	1.19 (0.53–2.66)	0.673
Diagnosis of chronic diseases (%)				
Cancer	92 (22.49)	156 (16.72)	1.48 (1.11–1.98)	0.008
Diabetes	108 (26.41)	146 (15.65)	1.90 (1.44–2.51)	<0.0001
COPD	166 (40.59)	244 (26.15)	2.01 (1.56–2.59)	<0.0001
End-stage renal disease	10 (2.44)	15 (1.61)	1.67 (0.75–3.72)	0.213

[a] Number (%) of patients or median (IQ); [b] OR calculated for 10-year increments; [c] OR calculated for 1000-DDD increments; [d] OR calculated for 10-day increments. Abbreviations: QREC = quinolone-resistant E. coli.

The univariate analysis showed that receiving at least one FQ prescription in the year preceding the diagnosis of resistance was associated with a higher risk of being colonized or infected with QREC (OR 3.87, 95% CI 2.88–5.18, $p < 0.0001$) than receiving an antibiotic prescription in the preceding 2nd year (OR 2.72, 95% CI 2.04–3.64, $p < 0.0001$) or in the preceding 3rd, 4th or 5th year (OR 1.90, 95% CI 1.49–2.44, $p < 0.0001$). Consistently, after adjustment for relevant confounding factors (age, gender, days of hospitalization and comorbidities (COPD and diabetes)), the risk of QREC colonization/infection was highest in the first year preceding the diagnosis of resistance (OR 2.67, 95% CI 1.92–3.70, $p < 0.0001$); then, it decreased progressively (OR 1.54, 95%CI 1.09–2.17, $p = 0.015$) to become undetectable after two years (OR 1.09, 95% CI 0.80–1.48, $p = 0.997$) (Table 2).

Table 2. Multivariable conditional logistic regression analysis focused on the association between previous FQ use and FQ resistance in E. coli over a five-year period.

Variable	Adjusted OR (95% CI)	p
At least one FQ prescription in 1st previous year	2.67 (1.92–3.70)	<0.0001
At least one FQ prescription taken in previous 2nd year	1.54 (1.09–2.17)	0.015
At least one FQ prescription taken in previous 3rd, 4th or 5th year	1.09 (0.80–1.48)	0.997
Age	1.09 [a] (1.01–1.18)	0.026
Gender, male	1.42 (1.07–1.88)	0.016
Hospitalization days	1.03 [b] (1.01–1.06)	0.022
Diagnosis of chronic diseasesDiabetes	1.41 (0.96–1.80)	0.037
COPD	1.43 (1.05–1.87)	0.019

[a] OR calculated for 10-year increments; [b] OR calculated for 10-day increments. Abbreviations: FQ = fluoroquinolone, COPD = chronic obstructive pulmonary disease.

In addition, the analysis showed that older age, male sex, longer hospital stays and being affected by diabetes mellitus and/or COPD are independent risk factors for FQ resistance in E. coli.

The multivariable analysis focused on FQ use in the 12 months preceding the diagnosis of resistance (Table 3) showed, consistently with the univariate analysis, that the use of FQs is strongly associated with FQ resistance in E. coli. After adjustment for relevant confounding factors and including exposure to any antibiotic other than FQs in the model, a clear dose–response effect could be observed: the use of FQs increases the risk of FQ resistance in E. coli more than fourfold if the patient was exposed to three or more courses of FQ in the previous 12 months (OR 4.21, 95% CI 2.38–7.50, $p < 0.0001$), and it decreases with lower cumulative exposures (OR 2.76, 95% CI 1.63–4.66, $p < 0.0001$ and 2.40, 95% CI 1.62–3.56, $p < 0.0001$ after two courses and one course of FQ in the previous 12 months, respectively).

Table 3. Multivariable conditional logistic regression analysis focused on the association between FQ use and FQ resistance in *E. coli* over a 12–month period (dose-response effect).

Variables	Adjusted OR (95%CI)	p
FQ prescription in previous year		
0	Ref.	Ref.
1	2.40 (1.62–3.56)	<0.0001
2	2.76 (1.63–4.66)	<0.0001
3+	4.21 (2.38–7.50)	<0.0001
At least one other J01 prescription in previous year	1.10 (0.83–1.45)	0.516
Age	1.11 [a] (1.03–1.20)	0.008
Gender	1.39 (1.05–1.84)	0.010
Hospitalization days	1.03 [b] (1.01–1.06)	0.020
Diagnosis of chronic diseases		
Diabetes	1.40 (1.02–1.93)	0.037
COPD	1.46 (1.09–1.96)	0.004

[a] OR calculated for 10-year increments; [b] OR calculated for 10-day increments. Abbreviations: FQ = fluoroquinolone, COPD = Chronic obstructive pulmonary disease.

The two sensitivity analyses that excluded patients with very recent antibiotic exposures (<15 days from the ID) and patients at risk for hospital-acquired infections showed results that were consistent with those of the main analyses (Tables S3 and S4 of Supplementary File).

3. Discussion

3.1. Summary of the Principal Findings

This matched case–control study is the first of its kind to use administrative and routinely collected clinical data—which characterize, in a large sample of patients, the impact of previous FQ use in primary care and QREC colonization/infection over a five-year period—in a multi-database approach. In general, the risk of developing a community-acquired QREC colonization/infection increases in all those patients who had received FQs. The risk of resistance is highest in the first year after the antibiotic is taken; afterwards, it decreases progressively, becoming undetectable after 24 months. In addition, the risk of resistance is higher after greater cumulative exposures. Apart from antibiotic use, older age, male sex, longer hospital stays, COPD and diabetes mellitus are independent risk factors for FQ resistance in *E. coli*.

3.2. Findings of the Present Study in Light of Previous Observations

Our findings are in accordance with those of previous observational studies. Costelloe [9] and Bhakit [8] reported a consistent amount of existing evidence of an association between the decrease in antibiotic use and the subsequent decrease in resistance. At the same time, the authors of these systematic reviews highlighted a lack of evidence regarding time intervals of more than 12 months between antibiotic use and the diagnosis of resistance. What our study adds is the finding that FQ resistance can last for up to 24 months after the selective pressure of antimicrobials is removed, a longer time than previously reported. With respect to this, Hammond et al. recently demonstrated an association between antibiotic dispensing reduction in primary care and a decrease in ciprofloxacin, trimethoprim and amoxicillin resistance in *E. coli* within the subsequent quarter [15]. In contrast to the approach used in the latter and in other studies, e.g., as in Cuevas et al. [16], we were able to quantify the impact on resistance of previous antibiotic use at an individual level, avoiding the risk of the so-called ecological fallacy. Some studies, also mostly ecological, showed persistent bacterial resistance despite reduced antibiotic use in *E. coli* and in other species [17,18], while other studies showed the opposite [10,19,20]. A possible explanation of these divergent findings is likely the fact that bacterial resistance is a complex phenomenon, with primary care prescribing being only one of its drivers [21]. Vellinga et al. compared the resistance of *E. coli* to trimethoprim and ciprofloxacin with prescriptions of these antimicrobials at the GP practice level. The authors reported that the risk of a QREC colonization/infection increased by 8% for every additional prescription of ciprofloxacin per 1000 patients [22]. Similar to what they found at a community level, we show a clear dose–response effect in the association between FQ use and FQ resistance.

A recent systematic review by Zhu et al. identified, among others, relevant risk factors for QREC colonization/infection as previous antibiotic use (OR 2.74, 95% CI 1.92–3.92), quinolones (OR 7.67, 95% CI 4.79–12.26), diabetes mellitus (OR 1.62, 95% CI 1.43–1.83), previous hospitalization (OR 2.06, 95% CI 1.62–2.60), male sex (OR 1.41, 95% CI 1.21–1.64) and organ transplantation (OR 2.37, 95% CI 1.17–4.79) [23]. Our results are in line with these findings with regard to the above-mentioned risk factors, except for organ transplantation (data not shown), probably due to the very low prevalence of this condition in our dataset. Zhu et al. reported that older age was not found to be a risk factor of QREC colonization/infection, differently than in the present study, although the authors hypothesized that heterogeneity among studies affected this finding. Furthermore, the study identified as significant risk factors for QREC colonization/infection the presence of a urinary catheter, urinary tract abnormalities and having had previous UTIs. We were not able to verify these associations because data on these conditions were not available to us. Nonetheless, in our case, the majority (i.e., 73%) of specimens that contributed to our study were urine samples. As we could demonstrate the reversibility of FQ resistance in *E. coli*, and taking into consideration that this species is the most common urinary pathogen [24], considered to be resistant to FQ in up to 40% of cases [14], antibiotic stewardship interventions seem well placed when directed to reduce antibiotic consumption for UTI, especially in primary care settings, as suggested elsewhere [25–28].

3.3. Strengths and Limitations of the Study

A strength of the present study is the comprehensiveness of the data source, namely, the database of the regional laboratories, the database of outpatient drug prescription records and the hospital discharge record databases.

We used data from the regional laboratories of the Autonomous Province of Bolzano to select cases that were matched to all available controls derived from the same data source. This assured comparability of cases and controls, as both were selected from the same source population, in which we did not assume the existence of any selection factor related to the exposure or outcome. Furthermore, comparability over time (namely, when the resistance was, or was not, diagnosed) was assured as we used the index date, namely, the date of the bacterial culture, as the matching variable.

The linkage of the above database with those containing the hospital discharge records and the outpatient drug prescription records is a further strength. The latter databases contain data from every single hospital discharge carried out in the given period and of any pharmaceutical prescription issued by primary care physicians in the whole catchment area and in the examined period. This allowed us to collect data on exposures from earlier years without the risk of recall bias that could lead to differential misclassification.

Nonetheless, some limitations have to be considered.

First, we had to restrict the analyses to only a few relevant comorbidities because data derived from the hospital discharge record database were incomplete. Therefore, we could not exclude residual confounding.

Second, our sample included only adult patients, which could limit our findings' generalizability to younger adults or children.

Third, in this study, we had information on the exact date of the diagnosis of resistance for both cases and controls, but it is possible that the outcome (namely, the onset of the resistance) preceded the exposure in some of the cases (reverse causality). For this reason, as in all case–control studies, interpreting the associations we found as causal should be carried out with caution. At the same time, it is likely that the risk of reverse causality is low in our case, as multiple bacterial cultures were carried out for many of the included patients, and the less recent was used to define the cases and controls.

Fourth, the DDD gives a rough estimate of drug consumption, dose and duration of the treatment.

Fifth, we assumed that the antibiotics prescribed were actually taken. This could have led to an overestimation of the exposure.

Finally, we had no information on privately purchased antibiotics in our sample, which could have led to a non-differential underestimation of the exposure. However, according to aggregated data published annually by the Italian Medicine Agency, in Italy, privately purchased FQs that cannot be tracked account for less than 2% of total outpatient antibiotic consumption [29].

3.4. Meaning of the Study and Implication for Practice and Policy

E. coli isolates from individual patients with previous primary care prescriptions of FQs are more likely to be resistant to FQs than those collected from patients without. A single course of FQ is sufficient to increase the risk of resistance for up to two years. The risk for a patient to carry FQ-resistant *E. coli* strains is higher with more courses of previously prescribed FQs. Primary care clinicians may consider these findings, consistent to current recommendations, as a further reason to avoid unnecessary FQ use whenever possible.

3.5. Implications for Future Research

The factors contributing to bacterial resistance to antimicrobials are diverse, with antibiotic prescribing in primary care being only one of its causes. Future studies should be designed to evaluate the individual risk of resistance of different bacterial species to different antibiotics, controlling, in a one-health perspective, also for additional factors other than primary care prescribing, such as prescribing in hospitals, wastewater treatment and intensive farming. Prospective designs, especially randomized controlled trials, rather than ecological studies, should be adopted to assess the impact of primary care antibiotic stewardship interventions on resistance rates of different bacterial species in individual patients over time to better assess causality.

4. Methods

4.1. Study Design, Setting and Data Sources

This case–control study was conducted in the Autonomous Province of Bolzano, which, on the date of 1 January 2016, accounted for 525,475 inhabitants [30]. As data sources, the following information systems were anonymously linked to each other:

- The database of hospital reference laboratories was used to define cases and controls.
- The database of outpatient pharmaceutical prescriptions was used to define the exposure.
- The hospital discharge record database was used to identify potential risk factors.

From the database of hospital laboratories, we extracted all patients admitted to one of the local hospitals in 2016 and for whom a bacterial culture test was carried out. Analyses were conducted on blood, urine, respiratory tract secretions, soft tissue specimens and other samples (including vulvar, vaginal and perianal specimens; ascites and other abdominal fluid; pleural liquid; and post-surgery drainage fluid). The VITEK II system (bioMérieux, Hazelwood, MO, USA) or Maldi-TOF was used to identify bacterial species, and VITEK II was also used to perform antibiotic susceptibility testing. Following the EUCAST expert rules, ciprofloxacin was used as indicator antibiotic to detect FQ resistance in *E. coli* [31]. The yearly updated EUCAST interpretation criteria (Available online: http://www.eucast.org/ (accessed on 12 May 2022)) were used to interpret antibiograms, and specimens were either classified as resistant (R), susceptible (S) or intermediate (I). Only patients carrying FQ R or S *E. coli* isolates were included in the study.

From the database of outpatient pharmaceutical prescriptions, we extracted all prescriptions issued from 1 January 2012 to 31 December 2016 by primary care physicians located in the Province of Bolzano (general practitioners and out of hours primary care physicians). We categorized antibiotics through the Anatomical Therapeutic Chemical (ATC) (Available online: https://www.whocc.no/ (accessed on 29 April 2022)) classification system (Supplementary File, Table S1) and used the cumulative defined daily doses (DDDs) of different drug classes prescribed in the five years preceding the "index date" (ID) as a comorbidity measure (Supplementary File, Table S2) [32,33].

From the hospital discharge records database, consistently with a recent literature review [23], we extracted the following potential confounding factors: age; gender; total days of hospitalizations; hospitalization with surgery, with device implantation or with organ transplant; and diagnosis of chronic diseases (cancer, diabetes, chronic obstructive pulmonary disease (COPD) and hemodialysis).

Potential confounding factors and their data sources are listed in Table 4.

Table 4. Potential risk factors for FQ resistance in *E. coli* and their data source.

Potential Confounding Factor	Data Source
Age	hospital discharge records database
Gender	hospital discharge records database
Drug's DDD taken in previous 5 years	database of drug prescription records
Number of active ingredients taken in previous 5 years	database of drug prescription records
Number of antibiotics taken in previous 5 years	database of drug prescription records
One or more J01 prescription taken in previous 5, 4 and 3 years	database of drug prescription records
One or more J01 prescription taken in previous 2 years	database of drug prescription records
Hospitalization days	hospital discharge records database
Hospitalizations	hospital discharge records database
Hospitalizations with surgery	hospital discharge records database
Hospitalizations with device implantation	hospital discharge records database
Hospitalizations with organ transplant	hospital discharge records database
Diagnosis of chronic diseases	hospital discharge records database
Cancer	
Diabetes Mellitus	
COPD	
Hemodialysis	

Abbreviations: DDD = defined daily dose; COPD = chronic obstructive pulmonary disorder.

4.2. Definition of Cases and Controls

Patients were classified as cases if they were diagnosed with FQ-resistant isolates or as controls if they were diagnosed with FQ-susceptible isolates. We matched all available controls to each case, using the ID as the matching variable, defined as the day (±30 days) on which the culture test results became available. If the ID was not available, data were excluded from the analysis. If, during 2016, a patient had more than one culture test result, the less recent one was included in the analyses. The flow of included cases and controls is outlined in Figure 1.

4.3. Definition of Exposure

We defined the exposure of interest as the use of any FQ for systemic use (ATC codes are listed in Table S1 of the Supplementary File), grouped in the following three categories: (1) use of one or more FQ for systemic use in the first year preceding the ID, (2) use of one or more FQ for systemic use in the second year preceding the ID, and (3) use of one or more FQ for systemic use three to five years preceding the ID. In order to calculate the dose–response effect, exposed subjects were considered only those to whom at least one FQ was prescribed in the year preceding the ID, taking the number of prescriptions into account (0, 1, 2, 3 or more).

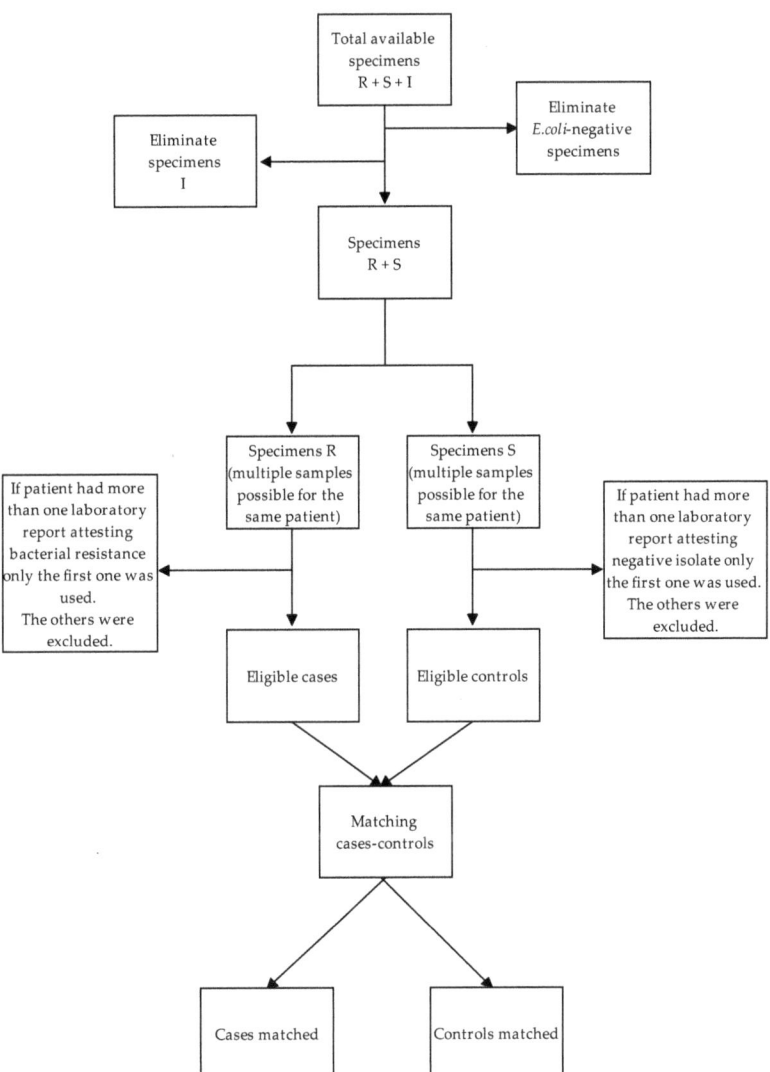

Figure 1. Flow of included cases and controls.

4.4. Statistical Analysis

We used descriptive statistics to compare the characteristics of included patients, presenting categorical variables as percentages and continuous variables as mean (± standard deviation) or, where appropriate, as median (interquartile range). We used univariate conditional logistic regression to assess the strength of the association between single independent variables and the outcome. We used matched odds ratios (ORs) and 95% confidence intervals (CIs) to evaluate the strength of any association. We considered those factors with p-values < 0.05 in the univariate analysis as eligible for inclusion in the multivariable models. Covariates to be included in the regression models were then selected using a backward stepwise approach.

4.5. Sensitivity Analyses

To evaluate the consistency of our results, we carried out the following sensitivity analyses: (a) in order to exclude all hospital-acquired infections from the outcome measure, we excluded from the analyses all patients with a culture carried out more than 48 h after their hospital admission; (b) in order to eliminate the effect of a very recent antibiotic use, we excluded all patients who received at least one prescription of antibiotics in the 15 days preceding the ID.

All the analyses were performed using STATA software package version 17.0 and R 3.6 [34,35].

Supplementary Materials: The following supporting information can be downloaded at: https://www.mdpi.com/article/10.3390/antibiotics11060822/s1, Table S1: Codes for exposure; Table S2: Codes for considered comorbidities; Table S3: Sensitivity analysis performed, excluding all patients who received at least one prescription of antibiotics in the 15 days preceding the ID; Table S4: Sensitivity analysis performed, excluding all patients with a bacterial culture performed after 48 h of hospital admission.

Author Contributions: Conceptualization, P.K.K., G.T., G.F. and M.M.; Data curation, P.K.K., C.F., R.D.C., G.F., R.A., V.M. and E.P.; Formal analysis, P.K.K., C.F., S.S.A. and M.M.; Investigation, P.K.K.; Methodology, P.K.K., C.F., G.T., G.F. and M.M.; Project administration, R.D.C., G.T. and M.M.; Supervision, G.T., O.M., I.G. and S.S.A.; Writing—original draft, P.K.K.; Writing—review and editing, P.K.K., C.F., R.D.C., O.M., I.G., R.A., S.S.A. and M.M. All authors have read and agreed to the published version of the manuscript.

Funding: This research received no external funding.

Institutional Review Board Statement: The study was conducted according to the Declaration of Helsinki and approved by the ethics committee of the Italian National Institute of Health (Istituto Superiore di Sanità, in-house protocol PRE-555/17—17 July 2017).

Informed Consent Statement: Waived due to the retrospective nature of the study performed on anonymous clinical data.

Data Availability Statement: Raw data are available upon reasonable request from the corresponding author.

Conflicts of Interest: The authors declare no conflict of interest.

References

1. Spellberg, B.; Bartlett, J.G.; Gilbert, D.N. The future of antibiotics and resistance. *N. Engl. J. Med.* **2013**, *368*, 299–302. [CrossRef]
2. Williams, D.N. Antimicrobial resistance: Are we at the dawn of the post-antibiotic era? *JR Coll. Physicians Edinb.* **2016**, *46*, 150–156. [CrossRef]
3. Murray, C.J.L.; Ikuta, K.S.; Sharara, F.; Swetschinski, L.; Robles Aguilar, G.; Gray, A.; Han, C.; Bisignano, C.; Rao, P.; Wool, E.; et al. Global burden of bacterial antimicrobial resistance in 2019: A systematic analysis. *Lancet* **2022**, *399*, 629–655. [CrossRef]
4. Review on Antimicrobial Resistance. Antimicrobial Resistance: Tackling a Crisis for the Health and Wealth of Nations. 2014. Available online: https://amr-review.org/sites/default/files/AMR%20Review%20Paper%20-%20Tackling%20a%20crisis%20for%20the%20health%20and%20wealth%20of%20nations_1.pdf (accessed on 4 April 2022).
5. World Health Organization. Global Action Plan on Antimicrobial Resistance. 2015. Available online: https://apps.who.int/iris/handle/10665/193736 (accessed on 4 April 2022).
6. Curtis, H.J.; Walker, A.J.; Mahtani, K.R.; Goldacre, B. Time trends and geographical variation in prescribing of antibiotics in England 1998–2017. *J. Antimicrob. Chemother.* **2019**, *74*, 242–250. [CrossRef] [PubMed]
7. Majeed, A.; Moser, K. Age- and sex-specific antibiotic prescribing patterns in general practice in England and Wales in 1996. *Br. J. Gen. Pract.* **1999**, *49*, 735–736.
8. Bakhit, M.; Hoffmann, T.; Scott, A.M.; Beller, E.; Rathbone, J.; Del Mar, C. Resistance decay in individuals after antibiotic exposure in primary care: A systematic review and meta-analysis. *BMC Med.* **2018**, *16*, 126. [CrossRef]
9. Costelloe, C.; Metcalfe, C.; Lovering, A.; Mant, D.; Hay, A.D. Effect of antibiotic prescribing in primary care on antimicrobial resistance in individual patients: Systematic review and meta-analysis. *BMJ* **2010**, *340*, c2096. [CrossRef]
10. Bryce, A.; Hay, A.D.; Lane, I.F.; Thornton, H.V.; Wootton, M.; Costelloe, C. Global prevalence of antibiotic resistance in paediatric urinary tract infections caused by Escherichia coli and association with routine use of antibiotics in primary care: Systematic review and meta-analysis. *BMJ* **2016**, *352*, i939. [CrossRef]

11. Fulgenzio, C.; Massari, M.; Traversa, G.; Da Cas, R.; Ferrante, G.; Aschbacher, R.; Moser, V.; Pagani, E.; Vestri, A.R.; Massidda, O.; et al. Impact of Prior Antibiotic Use in Primary Care on Escherichia coli Resistance to Third Generation Cephalosporins: A Case-Control Study. *Antibiotics* **2021**, *10*, 451. [CrossRef]
12. Schmiemann, G.; Gágyor, I.; Hummers-Pradier, E.; Bleidorn, J. Resistance profiles of urinary tract infections in general practice—An observational study. *BMC Urol.* **2012**, *12*, 33. [CrossRef]
13. Klingeberg, A.; Noll, I.; Willrich, N.; Feig, M.; Emrich, D.; Zill, E.; Krenz-Weinreich, A.; Kalka-Moll, W.; Oberdorfer, K.; Schmiemann, G.; et al. Antibiotic-Resistant E. coli in Uncomplicated Community-Acquired Urinary Tract Infection. *Dtsch. Ärzteblatt Int.* **2018**, *115*, 494–500. [CrossRef] [PubMed]
14. Stapleton, A.E.; Wagenlehner, F.M.E.; Mulgirigama, A.; Twynholm, M. Escherichia coli Resistance to Fluoroquinolones in Community-Acquired Uncomplicated Urinary Tract Infection in Women: A Systematic Review. *Antimicrob. Agents Chemother.* **2020**, *64*, e00862-20. [CrossRef] [PubMed]
15. Hammond, A.; Stuijfzand, B.; Avison, M.B.; Hay, A.D. Antimicrobial resistance associations with national primary care antibiotic stewardship policy: Primary care-based, multilevel analytic study. *PLoS ONE* **2020**, *15*, e0232903. [CrossRef]
16. Cuevas, O.; Oteo, J.; Lázaro, E.; Aracil, B.; de Abajo, F.; García-Cobos, S.; Ortega, A.; Campos, J. Significant ecological impact on the progression of fluoroquinolone resistance in Escherichia coli with increased community use of moxifloxacin, levofloxacin and amoxicillin/clavulanic acid. *J. Antimicrob. Chemother.* **2011**, *66*, 664–669. [CrossRef] [PubMed]
17. Sundqvist, M.; Geli, P.; Andersson, D.I.; Sjölund-Karlsson, M.; Runehagen, A.; Cars, H.; Abelson-Storby, K.; Cars, O.; Kahlmeter, G. Little evidence for reversibility of trimethoprim resistance after a drastic reduction in trimethoprim use. *J. Antimicrob. Chemother.* **2010**, *65*, 350–360. [CrossRef]
18. Enne, V.I.; Livermore, D.M.; Stephens, P.; Hall, L.M. Persistence of sulphonamide resistance in Escherichia coli in the UK despite national prescribing restriction. *Lancet* **2001**, *357*, 1325–1328. [CrossRef]
19. Aliabadi, S.; Anyanwu, P.; Beech, E.; Jauneikaite, E.; Wilson, P.; Hope, R.; Majeed, A.; Muller-Pebody, B.; Costelloe, C. Effect of antibiotic stewardship interventions in primary care on antimicrobial resistance of Escherichia coli bacteraemia in England 2013–18: A quasi-experimental, ecological, data linkage study. *Lancet Infect. Dis.* **2021**, *21*, 1689–1700. [CrossRef]
20. Livermore, D.M.; Hope, R.; Reynolds, R.; Blackburn, R.; Johnson, A.P.; Woodford, N. Declining cephalosporin and fluoroquinolone non-susceptibility among bloodstream Enterobacteriaceae from the UK: Links to prescribing change? *J. Antimicrob. Chemother.* **2013**, *68*, 2667–2674. [CrossRef]
21. Holmes, A.H.; Moore, L.S.; Sundsfjord, A.; Steinbakk, M.; Regmi, S.; Karkey, A.; Guerin, P.J.; Piddock, L.J. Understanding the mechanisms and drivers of antimicrobial resistance. *Lancet* **2016**, *387*, 176–187. [CrossRef]
22. Vellinga, A.; Murphy, A.W.; Hanahoe, B.; Bennett, K.; Cormican, M. A multilevel analysis of trimethoprim and ciprofloxacin prescribing and resistance of uropathogenic Escherichia coli in general practice. *J. Antimicrob. Chemother.* **2010**, *65*, 1514–1520. [CrossRef]
23. Zhu, D.-M.; Li, Q.-H.; Shen, Y.; Zhang, Q. Risk factors for quinolone-resistant Escherichia coli infection: A systematic review and meta-analysis. *Antimicrob. Resist. Infect. Control* **2020**, *9*, 11. [CrossRef] [PubMed]
24. Flores-Mireles, A.L.; Walker, J.N.; Caparon, M.; Hultgren, S.J. Urinary tract infections: Epidemiology, mechanisms of infection and treatment options. *Nat. Rev. Microbiol.* **2015**, *13*, 269–284. [CrossRef] [PubMed]
25. Hillier, S.; Roberts, Z.; Dunstan, F.; Butler, C.; Howard, A.; Palmer, S. Prior antibiotics and risk of antibiotic-resistant community-acquired urinary tract infection: A case-control study. *J. Antimicrob. Chemother.* **2007**, *60*, 92–99. [CrossRef]
26. Alam, M.F.; Cohen, D.; Butler, C.; Dunstan, F.; Roberts, Z.; Hillier, S.; Palmer, S. The additional costs of antibiotics and re-consultations for antibiotic-resistant Escherichia coli urinary tract infections managed in general practice. *Int. J. Antimicrob. Agents* **2009**, *33*, 255–257. [CrossRef] [PubMed]
27. Kaußner, Y.; Röver, C.; Heinz, J.; Hummers, E.; Debray, T.; Hay, A.; Heytens, S.; Vik, I.; Little, P.; Moore, M.; et al. Reducing antibiotic use in uncomplicated urinary tract infections in adult women: A systematic review and individual participant data meta-analysis. *Clin. Microbiol. Infect.* **2022**; in press.
28. Fraile Navarro, D.; Sullivan, F.; Azcoaga-Lorenzo, A.; Hernandez Santiago, V. Point-of-care tests for urinary tract infections: Protocol for a systematic review and meta-analysis of diagnostic test accuracy. *BMJ Open* **2020**, *10*, e033424. [CrossRef]
29. Osservatorio Nazionale sull'impiego dei Medicinali. *L'uso degli antibiotici in Italia. Rapporto Nazionale 2019*; Agenzia Italiana del Farmaco (AIFA): Roma, Italy, 2020.
30. Popolazione residente—2016. ASTAT Istituto Provinciale di Statistica. Provincia Autonoma di Bolzano—Alto Adige. Available online: https://astat.provinz.bz.it/barometro/upload/statistikatlas/it/atlas.html#!bev/wohnbevbdv/wohnbev (accessed on 20 January 2021).
31. EUCAST Expert rules in antimicrobial susceptibility testing, version 1. April 2008. Available online: https://www.eucast.org/fileadmin/src/media/PDFs/4ESCMID_Library/3Publications/EUCAST_Documents/Other_Documents/EUCAST_Expert_rules_final_April_20080407.pdf (accessed on 12 May 2022).
32. WHO Collaborating Centre for Drug Statistics Methodology. Anatomical Therapeutic Chemical (ATC) classification system: Guidelines for ATC classification and DDD assignment. Oslo: Norwegian Institute of Public Health. 2020. Available online: https://www.whocc.no/filearchive/publications/2020_guidelines_web.pdf (accessed on 6 September 2020).
33. International Classification of Diseases, 9th revision. *Clinical Modification*, 5th ed.; Medicode: Salt Lake City, UT, USA, 1995.

34. StataCorp. *Stata Statistical Software: Release 17*; StataCorp LLC.: College Station, TX, USA, 2021.
35. R Core Team. R: A Language and Environment for Statistical Computing [Internet], Vienna, Austria. 2016. Available online: https://www.R-project.org/ (accessed on 29 April 2022).

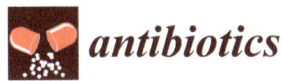

Article

The Impact of a Post-Prescription Review and Feedback Antimicrobial Stewardship Program in Lebanon

Anita Shallal [1], Chloe Lahoud [2], Dunia Merhej [3], Sandra Youssef [3], Jelena Verkler [1], Linda Kaljee [4], Tyler Prentiss [4], Seema Joshi [1], Marcus Zervos [1,5] and Madonna Matar [3,6,*]

1. Division of Infectious Diseases, Henry Ford Hospital, Detroit, MI 48202, USA; ashalla2@hfhs.org (A.S.); jverkle1@hfhs.org (J.V.); sjoshi5@hfhs.org (S.J.); mzervos1@hfhs.org (M.Z.)
2. Division of Infectious Diseases, Brigham & Women's Hospital, Harvard Medical School, Boston, MA 02115, USA; clahoud@bwh.harvard.edu
3. Notre Dame des Secours University Hospital, Byblos 1401, Lebanon; merhejdunia@gmail.com (D.M.); sandra.j.youssef@gmail.com (S.Y.)
4. Global Health Initiative, Henry Ford Hospital, Detroit, MI 48202, USA; lkaljee1@hfhs.org (L.K.); tprenti1@hfhs.org (T.P.)
5. Office of Global Affairs, Wayne State University School of Medicine, Detroit, MI 48202, USA
6. School of Medicine and Medical Sciences, Holy Spirit University of Kaslik, Byblos 1401, Lebanon
* Correspondence: madonnamatar@gmail.com

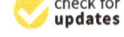

Citation: Shallal, A.; Lahoud, C.; Merhej, D.; Youssef, S.; Verkler, J.; Kaljee, L.; Prentiss, T.; Joshi, S.; Zervos, M.; Matar, M. The Impact of a Post-Prescription Review and Feedback Antimicrobial Stewardship Program in Lebanon. *Antibiotics* 2022, 11, 642. https://doi.org/10.3390/antibiotics11050642

Academic Editors: Gyöngyvér Soós and Ria Benkő

Received: 6 March 2022
Accepted: 9 May 2022
Published: 11 May 2022

Publisher's Note: MDPI stays neutral with regard to jurisdictional claims in published maps and institutional affiliations.

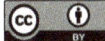

Copyright: © 2022 by the authors. Licensee MDPI, Basel, Switzerland. This article is an open access article distributed under the terms and conditions of the Creative Commons Attribution (CC BY) license (https://creativecommons.org/licenses/by/4.0/).

Abstract: Antimicrobial stewardship programs (ASPs) are effective means to optimize prescribing practices. They are under-utilized in the Middle East where many challenges exist for ASP implementation. We assessed the effectiveness of infectious disease physician-driven post-prescription review and feedback as an ASP in Lebanon. This prospective cohort study was conducted over an 18-month period in the medical, surgical, and intensive care units of a tertiary care hospital. It consisted of three phases: the baseline, intervention, and follow-up. There was a washout period of two months between each phase. Patients aged ≥16 years receiving 48 h of antibiotics were included. During the intervention phase, the AMS team reviewed antimicrobial use within 72 h post-prescription and gave alternate recommendations based on the guidelines for use. The acceptance of the recommendations was measured at 72 h. The primary outcome of the study was days of therapy per 1000 study patient days. A total of 328 patients were recruited in the baseline phase (August–October 2020), 467 patients in the intervention phase (January–June 2021), and 301 patients in the post-intervention phase (September–December 2021). The total days of therapy decreased from 11.46 during the baseline phase to 8.64 during the intervention phase ($p < 0.001$). Intervention acceptance occurred 88.5% of the time. The infectious disease physician-driven implementation of an ASP was successful in reducing antibiotic utilization in an acute care setting in Lebanon.

Keywords: global health; antimicrobial stewardship; COVID-19; disaster planning

1. Introduction

Antimicrobial resistance (AMR) is an urgent threat to global health; contributing to over 8 million hospital stays, it costs healthcare systems over USD 20 billion [1] and is anticipated to result in the death of 10 million people per year by 2050 [2,3]. AMR is a unique challenge, particularly in areas of the Middle East where health services have been severely impacted by conflict [4]. In these collapsed health systems, there may be a lack of laboratories and other diagnostic tools amidst the unregulated use of antibiotics [4]. In one observational study, multidrug-resistant organisms were frequently detected in water in Lebanon, serving as a potential reservoir for the dissemination of resistant organisms [5]. Furthermore, conflict contributes to a shortage of healthcare providers, further worsening the overall crisis [6]. The lack of overall data and surveillance of AMR in this region makes it especially difficult to compare it with the rest of the world, thus limiting opportunities for intervention. More recently, barriers for the region were summarized and included a need for the training of healthcare personnel and an increased laboratory capacity for the surveillance of AMR as well as the development of antimicrobial stewardship (AMS) guidelines [7].

The most important causes of AMR are inappropriate antimicrobial prescribing and use [2]. Recognizing the urgency of this issue, various AMS programs (ASPs) have been implemented to reduce AMR and promote proper prescribing practices. In order for ASPs to be effective, significant infrastructural components must be present, including national and institutional prescribing policies, healthy prescriber–pharmacist relationships, surveillance and reviews of prescribing practices, and stakeholder buy-ins [8]. Institutions in the Middle East are lacking in firm guidelines for proper antimicrobial use. One systematic review identified 20 studies that described potential proactive interventions with impacts on the de-escalation of antibiotics, discontinuation rates of restricted antibiotics, and length of hospital stay, and that prospective audits and feedback were beneficial for the clinical outcome [1]. Yet, it was also noted that cultural considerations in the Middle East such as physician attitudes, the acceptance of collaborative practices, and the acceptance of pharmacist recommendations may limit effectiveness [1].

The post-prescription review and feedback (PPRF) program has been shown to be effective in the United States and in low- to middle-income countries, including Nepal and India [9–11]. This method of ASP has not been demonstrated to be effective in the Middle East and North Africa regions. This project evaluated the impact of a PPRF program at a tertiary hospital in Lebanon.

2. Materials and Methods

2.1. Study Design and Setting

This prospective cohort study was carried out to determine the feasibility of the implementation of an ASP. The study period consisted of 21 months from April 2020 to December 2021, and was divided into 3 phases: the baseline (3 months), intervention (6 months), and post-intervention (4 months). There was a washout period of 2 months between each phase. The project was a collaboration between the Henry Ford Hospital Division of Infectious Diseases (Detroit, MI, USA) and Notre Dame des Secours University Hospital (Byblos, Lebanon). The Notre Dame des Secours University Hospital is a private, not-for-profit tertiary care teaching hospital with 242 beds and covers a diverse population of medical cases from a wide geographic area. For the present study, the PPRF program was piloted in medicine, surgery, and intensive care unit wards.

In this institution, there was no integrated multidisciplinary AMS team. A team was established to supervise and complete all phases of the project. The dedicated AMS team was composed of an ID specialist, and infection prevention and control officers. The institutional review boards of Notre Dame des Secours University Hospital and Henry Ford Hospital approved the study. A waiver of consent was obtained due to the nature of the study.

2.2. Identification of the Study Participants

Participants were selected from medical, surgical, and intensive care unit wards and were managed by a primary treating team who remained the same throughout the study. The inclusion criteria were that all patients were aged ≥ 16 years and had received antibiotics for ≥ 48 h. The exclusion criteria were patients aged ≤ 16 years and on antibiotics for ≤ 48 h. All medical and surgical specialties were included in the study and patients fulfilling the eligibility criteria were recruited daily. The medical records were reviewed and data were collected at each phase of the study, including the demographic data (age and gender), comorbidity, infection type, antibiotic used, length of hospital stay, and total antibiotic days.

2.3. Design of the Phases and the Evaluation of Antimicrobial Use

The baseline phase involved 3 months of evaluation of antimicrobial therapy without the provision of any recommendations. Meanwhile, continuous education was initiated and included regional AMR data and the prevention and management of resistance as well as the components and goals of the ASP, details regarding the PPRF implementation within the institution, and a review of the medical guidelines. Sessions were delivered to physicians in different specialties. Practice guidelines were prepared and supervised by the ID specialist and sent to all physicians working at the institution. The guidelines contained recommendations for an empiric therapy (given for early sepsis with an unclear etiology) as well as a definitive therapy for common infectious syndromes, intravenous to oral conversions, renal-adjusted dosing, and the duration of the antibiotic therapy. Due to the COVID-19 pandemic, webinars were scheduled to educate the healthcare staff and address questions regarding these topics.

The intervention phase occurred following a 2-month washout period. The phase consisted of 6 months of intervention, during which the AMS team initiated a consultation for all eligible patients. During the AMS consultation, the ID physician was responsible for informing the primary treatment team of any recommendations about an antibiotic change. Types of interventions included dose optimization, the escalation of therapy, the de-escalation of therapy, route changes, drug discontinuation, the optimization of administration modalities, and "other". The final decision to act on the recommendations was left to the primary team. The willingness to accept the intervention, type of primary service, and reasons for not accepting the intervention were also recorded ("not convinced", "felt insecure", or "needed a longer duration"). For this study, "not convinced" implied that they were not convinced by the AMS team to accept the recommendation and "felt insecure" implied a lack of confidence in changing antimicrobials.

The final (post-intervention) phase occurred after a 2-month washout period. It was designed to re-assess antibiotic prescriptions in the same way as the baseline phase for a period of 4 months to assess if the ASP could be sustained without an intervention. During each period, AMS education continued via webinars, facility-based guidelines, and emails.

2.4. Outcome Measures

The primary outcome measure was the antimicrobial DOT at the baseline, intervention, and post-intervention phases. In this study, patient antibiotic days included the day on which the treatment with the antibiotic began through the stoppage of the drug or hospital discharge. Additionally, information regarding the class/type of antibiotic utilized in each phase and for what illness was also compared. The patient-specific outcome was the length of hospital stay per phase.

At the time of the PPRF launch, an email was sent to all physicians within the hospital introducing the ASP. A survey was prepared and sent by email to all 106 physicians in the institution admitting patients to the 3 mentioned units to evaluate the qualitative data, including the perceptions and attitudes regarding antibiotics, level of basic knowledge about antibiotic prescriptions and resistance, and outcome data that could be used to identify potential barriers and facilitators in the implementation and dissemination of future ASPs.

2.5. Statistical Analysis

Continuous data were described using means and standard deviations whereas categorical data were described using counts and column percentages. Univariate two-group comparisons were conducted using independent two-group *t*-tests for the continuous variables and chi-squared tests for the categorical variables. Two Poisson regression models were utilized to assess the magnitude and significance of the intervention phase on antibiotic days and hospitalization treatment days whilst adjusting for the confounders of age, gender, and treatment indication category. The total DOT per 1000 study patient days (PDs) was calculated at the baseline, intervention, and post-intervention periods for each antibiotic. An ANOVA was used to compare the mean antibiotics per day between the phases. The proportion of each variable was compared between the baseline and intervention time points, then between the intervention and post-intervention time points, then between the baseline and post-intervention periods using tests of proportion. These values were then compared using proportion tests with a Bonferroni adjustment between the phases. The statistical significance was set at $p < 0.05$. The analyses were performed using Epi Info-7 (Centers for Disease Control and Prevention, Atlanta, GA, USA) and SAS 9.4 (SAS Institute Inc., Cary, NC, USA).

3. Results

3.1. Study Population

A total of 328 patients were recruited in the baseline phase (August–October 2020), 467 patients in the intervention phase (January–June 2021), and 301 patients in the post-intervention phase (September–December 2021) (Table 1). There was an even distribution of gender across the baseline and intervention, but significantly more females in the post-intervention period ($p = 0.045$). The mean age of patients was 67.6 years in the baseline group; patients were significantly younger in the intervention group compared with pre-intervention, which occurred in a COVID-19 surge ($p = 0.002$). In the baseline period, compared with both the intervention and post-intervention periods, there were significantly more patients with pulmonary comorbidities (32% vs. 6.2% vs. 6.9%, $p < 0.001$). There were significantly more patients with a hepatic/gastrointestinal comorbidity in the intervention and post-intervention periods when compared with the baseline period (1.5% vs. 4.9% vs. 4.7%, $p = 0.01$). Oncologic and renal diseases were significantly more common in the post-intervention period (17.8%, $p = 0.001$ and 14.5%, $p = 0.002$, respectively).

Table 1. Summary of demographic data and days of therapy.

Demographics	Pre-Intervention ($n = 328$)	Intervention ($n = 467$)	Post-Intervention ($n = 301$)	p-Value [a] Phase 1 vs. 2 [b] Phase 1 vs. 3 [c] Phase 2 vs. 3
Gender, female	40.24% (132)	38.89 (182)	46.48% (99)	0.69 [a], 0.05 [b], 0.08 [c]
Mean age (SD)	67.6 (16.7) Range 17–97	63.72 (17.65) Range 16–96	65.84 (17.4) Range 16–97	<0.01 [a], 0.02 [b], 0.10 [c]
Median LOS (SD)	6.00 (6.7) Range 1–41	6.00 (4.8) Range 1–42	7.00 (5.1) Range 3–75	<0.01
Median duration of antibiotic course	5.00 (6.27) Range 1–40	5.00 (4.26) Range 1–39	6.00 (5.01) Range 2–25	<0.01
Median duration of antibiotic days/patient (SD)	8.00 (12.44) Range 1–118	7.00 (7.4) Range 1–63	8.0 (9.46) Range 1–63	<0.01
Pulmonary	32.01% (105)	6.21% (29)	6.9% (21)	<0.01 [a], <0.01 [b], 0.70 [c]
Cardiac	51.83% (170)	52.68% (246)	48.7% (148)	0.81 [a], 0.43 [b], 0.29 [c]
Vascular	3.05% (10)	1.93% (9)	2.6% (8)	0.31 [a], 0.74 [b], 0.50 [c]
Endocrine	35.98% (118)	39.4% (184)	35.5% (108)	0.33 [a], 0.90 [b], 0.29 [c]
Neurologic	5.79% (19)	7.49% (35)	4.6% (14)	0.35 [a], 0.50 [b], 0.11 [c]
Hepatic/GI	1.52% (5)	4.93% (23)	3.9% (12)	0.01 [a], 0.06 [b], 0.53 [c]
Heme/onc	9.15% (30)	14.99% (70)	17.8% (54)	0.01 [a], <0.01 [b], 0.29 [c]
Renal	7.01% (23)	8.57% (40)	14.47% (44)	0.42 [a], <0.01 [b], 0.01 [c]
Other	6.71% (22)	16.9% (79)	19.1% (58)	<0.01 [a], <0.01 [b], 0.43 [c]

3.2. Evaluation of Antimicrobial Use

The type of infection treated varied considerably between the phases. However, across all 3 phases, the most common infection treated was pneumonia. In the intervention phase, there was a significantly higher number of patients receiving an empirical treatment (17.5% compared with 3.1% at the baseline, $p < 0.001$); this was also true for the post-intervention phase (7.6%, $p < 0.001$). The number of patients treated for a gastrointestinal infection or a urinary tract infection and receiving postoperative prophylaxis significantly decreased in the intervention and post-intervention phases and was most significant between the baseline and intervention phases (13.2% vs. 3.8%, $p < 0.001$; 25.1% vs. 13.5%, $p < 0.001$; and 11.1% vs. 4.1%, $p < 0.001$, respectively). Skin and soft tissue infections were significantly more common in the post-intervention phase (11.1% vs. 2.6% in intervention, $p < 0.004$).

In the intervention phase, which occurred during a COVID-19 surge, empiric therapies (3.1% vs. 17.5%, $p < 0.001$) and "other" infections (9.45% vs. 31.8%, $p < 0.001$) significantly increased (Table 2).

Table 2. Type of infection treated in each phase.

Treatment Indication	Pre-Intervention ($n = 326$)	Intervention ($n = 467$)	Post-Intervention ($n = 301$)	p-Value [a] Phase 1 vs. 2 [b] Phase 1 vs. 3 [c] Phase 2 vs. 3
Empirical treatment	3.07% (10)	17.5% (82)	7.6% (23)	<0.001 [a], 0.01 [b], 0.001 [c]
Pneumonia	26.69% (87)	23.3% (109)	22% (67)	0.276 [a], 0.17 [b] 0.69 [c]
Gastrointestinal	13.19% (43)	3.85% (18)	3.9% (12)	<0.001 [a], <0.001 [b] 0.94 [c]
Sepsis	3.05% (10)	1.92% (9)	2.3% (7)	0.298 [a], 0.55 [b], 0.71 [c]
Urinary tract infection	25.15% (82)	13.46% (63)	18.1% (55)	<0.001 [a], 0.03 [b], 0.08 [c]
Postoperative prophylaxis	11.04% (36)	4.06% (19)	2.9% (9)	0.001 [a], 0.001 [b], 0.42 [c]
Skin and tissue infection	4.91% (16)	2.56% (12)	11.1% (34)	0.0784 [a], 0.004 [b], <0.0001 [c]
Diabetic foot infection	3.37% (11)	1.5% (7)	1.3% (4)	0.080 [a], 0.09 [b], 0.83 [c]
Other	9.45% (31)	31.8% (149)	32.9% (100)	<0.001 [a], <0.001 [b], 0.76 [c]

The choice of antimicrobial agent also significantly differed between the phases. There was an increase in days of vancomycin use compared with the baseline (57.83 DOT/1000 PD vs. 101.03, $p < 0.01$), with higher results in the post-intervention period compared with the baseline (150.26, $p < 0.01$). There was a significant reduction in the use of carbapenems between the baseline and intervention periods (455.62 DOT/1000 PD vs. 322.75, $p < 0.01$) with an increase in post-intervention prescribing in both phases (567.02 DOT/1000 PD, $p < 0.01$, $p < 0.01$). Beta-lactam use increased during the intervention phase (139.23 DOT/1000 PD to 187.24, $p < 0.01$) and returned to similar levels during post-intervention (122.97 DOT/1000 PD, $p < 0.01$) when compared with the intervention phase. In the post-intervention period, an increase in cephalosporin and carbapenem use was noted when compared with the baseline period; however, this did not reach a statistical significance. There was also a significant increase in the duration of aminoglycoside use in the post-intervention period when compared with the intervention period (4.6 vs. 2.9, $p = 0.004$) (Table 3).

Table 3. Antibiotic agent used in each phase.

DOT/1000 by Agent Mean	Baseline ($n = 328$, Patient Days 2715)	Intervention ($n = 467$, Patient Days 3306)	Post-Intervention ($n = 301$, Patient Days 2529)	p-Value [a] Phase 1 vs. 2 [b] Phase 1 vs. 3 [c] Phase 2 vs. 3
Intravenous antibiotics	1317.86	1205.08	1296.56	0.82
	1250.18	1197.96	1263.3	
Oral antibiotics	67.03	18.15	25.32	<0.01 [a], <0.01 [b], 0.06 [c]
Vancomycin	57.83	101.03	150.26	<0.01 [a], <0.01 [b], <0.01 [c]
Linezolid	15.84	11.8	22.14	0.53 [a], 0.28 [b], <0.01 [c]
Trimethoprim-sulfamethoxazole	11.42	0	0	<0.01 [a], <0.01 [b]
Doxycycline	7	0	1.98	<0.01 [a], 0.02 [b], 0.03 [c]
Penicillin	6.26	2.12	17	0.03 [a], <0.01 [b], <0.01 [c]
Beta-lactam/BLI	139.23	187.24	122.97	<0.01 [a], 0.25 [b], <0.01 [c]
Cephalosporin	306.08	399.58	248.71	<0.01 [a], <0.01 [b], <0.01 [c]
Carbapenem	455.62	322.75	567.02	<0.01 [a], <0.01 [b], <0.01 [c]
Metronidazole	60.77	51.72	27.68	0.38 [a], <0.01 [b], <0.01 [c]
Azithromycin	2.94	9.68	5.54	0.04 [a], 0.42 [b], 0.22 [c]
Clindamycin	2.58	9.98	17	<0.01 [a], <0.01 [b], 0.06 [c]
Fluoroquinolone	95.03	88.02	67.62	1.000 [a], <0.01 [b], <0.01 [c]
Colistin	0	0	25.3	<0.01 [b], <0.01 [c]
Aminoglycoside	20.99	11.19	16.2	0.01 [a], 0.6 [b], 0.29 [c]
Tigecycline	13.26	25.11	18.2	<0.01 [a], 0.45 [b], 0.23 [c]
Other	189.3	0	9.49	<0.01 [a], <0.01 [b], <0.01 [c]

BLI: beta-lactamase inhibitor; SD: standard deviation.

3.3. Intervention Acceptance

In the intervention phase, there were 467 interventions from the AMS team, which were accepted 414 times (88.5%). The most commonly performed intervention was "other" (234 (56.2%)), followed by drug discontinuation (108 (25.9%)). The escalation of therapy and the de-escalation of therapy occurred 25 times, respectively (6.1%, respectively). Dose optimization, route change, and administration modality optimization were less frequently performed (17 (4%), 5 (1.2%), and 2 (0.5%), respectively). For the 54 occurrences where an intervention was not accepted (11.5%), the reason for not accepting was most commonly due to a report of being "not convinced" (41 (75.9%)). Feeling insecure and needing a longer duration of therapy were less common reasons of not accepting (5 (9%) and 9 (16%), respectively). Among the types of interventions, the intervention that was most commonly not accepted was drug discontinuation (24%). Among the treatment providers, the primary service that did not accept an intervention the most frequently was surgery (15.9%) compared with medicine (12.4%) and the intensive care unit (12%).

3.4. Clinical Outcomes

Despite the increase in antimicrobial prescriptions for "other" infections and empirical therapies, the total days of antibiotic therapy decreased from 11.46 during the baseline phase to 8.64 days during the intervention phase ($p < 0.00001$). In the post-intervention phase, the total antibiotic days of therapy (DOT) was 10.9, and, although this number was lower than in the baseline phase, the effect did not meet a statistical significance ($p = 0.57$) (Table 1). After adjusting for age, sex, and treatment indication, members in the pre-intervention phase were on antibiotics 29% longer ($p < 0.001$) and hospitalized 16% longer ($p < 0.001$) than members in the intervention phase. After adjusting for age, sex, and treatment indication, members in the pre-intervention phase were on antibiotics 6% longer ($p = 0.02$) and hospitalized 3% longer ($p = 0.33$) than members in the post-intervention phase.

Of the 106 physicians, 20 completed the post-intervention survey, which was a response rate of 18.8%. The majority of respondents (12 (60%)) were female and the median age was 29.6 years old. Most respondents were practicing in the field of medicine (n = 14) and had a median of 6 years since the completion of their highest education. Their perceptions on antibiotic prescribing and knowledge were then assessed. The majority of respondents agreed or strongly agreed that inappropriate antibiotic prescribing put patients at risk and that AMR was a problem in the hospital where they worked. The majority of respondents felt that they had received inadequate training in antibiotic prescribing and that there was a need to increase the education of healthcare providers on AMR and antimicrobial prescribing. The majority of respondents felt that the PPRF would increase AMS without being disruptive to their work. Most respondents noted that they had never prescribed antibiotics because a patient insisted on it or to improve relationships with their patients. The most useful means of increasing antimicrobial prescribing education were felt to be short written guidelines, seminars, and summary written materials (Supplementary Tables S1–S4).

4. Discussion
4.1. PPRF Programs

This study was the first in Lebanon to examine the impact of the implementation of an infectious disease (ID) physician-driven PPRF strategy of AMS. In the intervention period, there was a significant reduction in DOT, type of illness treated, and types of antimicrobials in use and an indirect decrease in the length of hospital stay. The PPRF was noted to have many advantages. The program engaged the treating physicians with medical discussions, promoting an opportunity for education within medical teams. It also had a positive impact on collaborative clinical decision-making regarding antibiotic therapy modifications or discontinuations. Studies have shown that PPRFs build trust and rapport between treatment teams [11] with an associated decrease in DOT [12]. In addition, there is an opportunity for the AMS team to evaluate the barriers and enablers that can be used to modify the ASP [13]. At this institution, the PPRF was shown to be effective by not only decreasing the total DOT, but also by reducing the use of broad-spectrum antimicrobials such as carbapenems and beta-lactam/beta-lactamase inhibitors. The ASP had an indirect impact on the length of hospital stay of the patients, which was shorter in the intervention phase after adjusting for age, sex, and the treatment indication. Given that COVID-19 pandemic waves occurred in that time period, this could have been a bias that was not accounted for. However, this reduced length of hospital stay as a result of the ASP has also been noted in other studies [14].

Notably, the acceptance of the AMS team recommendations was 88%, which was higher than in prior studies that typically noted an acceptance rate of 60–70% [11,15,16]. We believed that the type of patients admitted (the majority was pneumonia, particularly given the COVID-19 surge in the intervention phase) and the use of verbal feedback and discussions as well as the continued stream of educational materials throughout the three phases of the study may have had an impact on the acceptance of recommendations. Additionally, the intervention was ID physician-led rather than pharmacist-led, as prior studies in the Middle East have noted less acceptance from pharmacists [15]. The most frequent reason for not accepting recommendations was the feeling of being "not convinced", which implied that there may be further work to be undertaken with further education on antibiotics with teams. Importantly, it is worth noting that feeling "not convinced" may actually relate to a need for behavioral change, with less reliance on personal knowledge or experience and more reliance on guidelines and formal policy [16,17]. Acceptance rates in this study were notably lower among surgical specialties, which was consistent with a prior similar study in Nepal [9]. Management guidelines across different specialties could strengthen the treating of the certainty of the clinical decisions of physicians, particularly when there are unified treatment algorithms according to local epidemiology data [18]. Furthermore, the integration of rapid diagnostic tools and the strengthening of laboratory capacities could help clinicians in their decision-making when empirically treating complicated cases [19].

4.2. Physician Attitudes

This study took into account the attitudes toward the ASP of the treating physicians at the study hospital. Although the number of participants in the survey was low, there was a general consensus among the participants about perceptions and barriers toward a PPRF. Additionally, the survey responses alerted a potential lack of confidence in knowledge about antibiotic prescribing and issues with insufficient training. The need for regular educational programs on prescribing has been cited in other ASPs [20]. Potential options for educational programs could include workshops and guidelines; prescribers tend to prefer guidelines locally developed rather than nationally developed [16]. Continued medical education should include seminars and modules with case studies and these educational programs should be routinely audited to ensure they can be integrated into prescriber schedules [9]. Importantly, three participants in the survey felt that the PPRF could be disruptive to the patient treatment. A recent study, also in Lebanon, evaluated physician attitudes toward the core elements of an ASP and found that 34% of participants felt that the ASP could affect physician autonomy [21]. Less restrictive stewardship programs, including PPRFs and antibiotic rounds, are possible ways to circumvent this issue, which may stem from cultural aspects of medicine in the region [15,22].

4.3. Impact of the Timeline on the Study

The study timeline directly coincided with COVID-19 surges that impacted on each phase. Two-month washouts were performed due to delays from the impact of COVID-19 and the economic collapse. Due to the increased hospitalization rate of COVID-19 patients, many were admitted to floors that were part of the intervention phase of the study and thus included in the PPRF. Admitted COVID-19 patients were frequently empirically treated for pneumonia, providing a unique opportunity for the AMS team to intervene, given prior studies that showed that although more than 90% of hospitalized COVID-19 patients received empiric antibiotics, only 15% were documented to have a secondary bacterial infection [23,24]. The rates were lower in other observational reports, increasing the hospital stay from 3.2% up to 6.1% [25]. However, it was unclear whether the COVID-19 surges in this study also led to greater antibiotic de-escalation as well as more readily acceptable interventions from our AMS team as a result of the known (viral-etiology) pandemic.

The economic collapse of Lebanon—which began in October 2019, but has significantly progressed since then (6)—directly impacted on the post-intervention phase of this study. During the post-intervention phase, there was a severe shortage of many antibiotics. Antibiotics were thus selected based on availability and not per empiric or treatment guidelines. This was clearly noted in our results where the use of carbapenems, cephalosporins, aminoglycosides, and colistin were higher in the post-intervention period. During this phase, an emphasis on the duration of therapy rather than the antibiotic agent choice was placed within stewardship education.

4.4. Strengths and Limitations

Separate from the direct impact of the economic collapse and COVID-19, there were other limitations to our study. Logistic challenges in place resulted in shortages of providers, which may have affected the ease of education of the treatment teams. Additionally, we did not take into account the severity of disease, mortality/survival benefit, or types of multidrug-resistant organisms treated, which might have impacted on the acceptance rate of the interventions, the type of interventions, and the type of antibiotics used. Finally, due to delays, the study was limited to an 18-month period, making assessments of changes to the AMR and susceptibility patterns impossible. This was also compounded by factors outside the control of a hospital program such as outpatient antimicrobials and antibiotic use in agricultural feeds.

A number of strengths exist in this study. First, the large number of patients recruited helped power the study appropriately for the analysis. Furthermore, the interrupted time series with washout periods between the phases reduced any bias that may have been associated with recent and direct education provided by the AMS team. Finally, the interventions were made with active dialogue and constant interaction with the treatment teams. This may have accounted for the increased acceptance of the recommendations compared with those PPRFs that use electronic medical record alerts. Using multidisciplinary collaboration and education were essential components of the ASP. Although labor-intensive, the overall primary outcome was clear and the secondary impact on the cost analysis given the reduction in the length of hospital stay is a potential direction for future studies.

5. Conclusions

Multifaceted approaches are needed to combat AMR across the Middle East. AMS education and strategies, including PPRFs, are useful methods to reduce DOT.

Supplementary Materials: The following supporting information can be downloaded at: https://www.mdpi.com/article/10.3390/antibiotics11050642/s1, Table S1: Physician survey responses—basic demographics.; Table S2: Physician survey responses on perceptions, knowledge, systemic failures and barriers, and attitudes towards a post-prescription review and feedback program (n = 20).; Table S3: Physician survey responses on supports and rewards for antimicrobial stewardship.; Table S4: Physician survey responses on useful means of increasing healthcare provider knowledge about antimicrobial resistance and treatment practices.

Author Contributions: A.S.—manuscript writing and editing, project analysis. C.L.—manuscript editing, project implementation. D.M.—concept development, project implementation. S.Y.—concept development, project implementation. J.V.—project analysis. L.K.—grant procurement, concept development. T.P.—grant procurement, concept development. S.J.—project analysis. M.Z.—grant procurement, concept development, manuscript editing. M.M.—grant procurement, concept development, manuscript writing and editing, project implementation. All authors have read and agreed to the published version of the manuscript.

Funding: Funding for this project was provided by Pfizer Global Medical Grants, #56142641.

Institutional Review Board Statement: The study was conducted in accordance with the Declaration of Helsinki, and approved/exempt for IRB review by Henry Ford Institutional Review Board under quality improvement (#14732), as well as exempt/approved under quality improvement through Notre Dame des Secours Institutional Review Board and Ethics Committee (#41735351).

Informed Consent Statement: Not applicable.

Data Availability Statement: Not applicable.

Conflicts of Interest: The authors declare no conflict of interest.

References

1. Nasr, Z.; Paravattil, B.; Wilby, K.J. The impact of antimicrobial stewardship strategies on antibiotic appropriateness and prescribing behaviours in selected countries in the Middle East: A systematic review. *East. Mediterr. Health J.* **2017**, *23*, 430–440. [CrossRef] [PubMed]
2. Ababneh, M.A.; Nasser, S.A.; Rababa'h, A.M. A systematic review of Antimicrobial Stewardship Program implementation in Middle Eastern countries. *Int. J. Infect. Dis.* **2021**, *105*, 746–752. [CrossRef] [PubMed]
3. Majumder, M.A.A.; Rahman, S.; Cohall, D.; Bharatha, A.; Singh, K.; Haque, M.; Gittens-St Hilaire, M. Antimicrobial stewardship: Fighting antimicrobial resistance and protecting global public health. *Infect. Drug Resist.* **2020**, *13*, 4713–4738. [CrossRef] [PubMed]
4. Devi, S. AMR in the Middle East: "A perfect storm". *Lancet* **2019**, *394*, 1311–1312. [CrossRef]
5. Moussa, J.; Abboud, E.; Tokajian, S. The dissemination of antimicrobial resistance determinants in surface water sources in Lebanon. *FEMS Microbiol. Ecol.* **2021**, *97*, fiab113. [CrossRef]
6. Shallal, A.; Lahoud, C.; Zervos, M.; Matar, M. Lebanon is losing its front line. *J. Glob. Health* **2021**, *11*, 03052. [CrossRef]
7. Al Salman, J.; Al Dabal, L.; Bassetti, M.; Alfouzan, W.A.; Al Maslamani, M.; Alraddadi, B.; Elhoufi, A.; Khamis, F.; Mokkadas, E.; Romany, I.; et al. Promoting cross-regional collaboration in antimicrobial stewardship: Findings of an infectious diseases working group survey in Arab countries of the Middle East. *J. Infect. Public Health* **2021**, *14*, 978–984. [CrossRef]
8. Goldmann, D.A.; Weinstein, R.A.; Wenzel, R.P.; Tablan, O.C.; Duma, R.J.; Gaynes, R.P.; Schlosser, J.; Martone, W.J. Strategies to prevent and control the emergence and spread of antimicrobial-resistant microorganisms in hospitals. A challenge to hospital leadership. *JAMA* **1996**, *275*, 234–240. [CrossRef]
9. Joshi, R.D.; Zervos, M.; Kaljee, L.M.; Shrestha, B.; Maki, G.; Prentiss, T.; Bajracharya, D.; Karki, K.; Joshi, N.; Rai, S.M. Evaluation of a hospital-based post-prescription review and feedback pilot in Kathmandu, Nepal. *Am. J. Trop. Med. Hyg.* **2019**, *101*, 923–928. [CrossRef]
10. Nauriyal, V.; Rai, S.M.; Joshi, R.D.; Thapa, B.B.; Kaljee, L.; Prentiss, T.; Maki, G.; Shrestha, B.; Bajracharya, D.C.; Karki, K.; et al. Evaluation of an antimicrobial stewardship program for wound and burn care in three hospitals in Nepal. *Antibiotics* **2020**, *9*, 914. [CrossRef]
11. Rupali, P.; Palanikumar, P.; Shanthamurthy, D.; Peter, J.V.; Kandasamy, S.; Zacchaeus, N.G.P.; Alexander, H.; Thangavelu, P.; Karthik, R.; Abraham, O.C.; et al. Impact of an antimicrobial stewardship intervention in India: Evaluation of post-prescription review and feedback as a method of promoting optimal antimicrobial use in the intensive care units of a tertiary-care hospital. *Infect. Control Hosp. Epidemiol.* **2019**, *40*, 512–519. [CrossRef]
12. Tamma, P.D.; Avdic, E.; Keenan, J.F.; Zhao, Y.; Anand, G.; Cooper, J.; Dezube, R.; Hsu, S.; Cosgrove, S.E. What is the more effective antibiotic stewardship intervention: Preprescription authorization or postprescription review with feedback? *Clin. Infect. Dis.* **2017**, *64*, 537–543.
13. Chavada, R.; Walker, H.N.; Tong, D.; Murray, A. Changes in antimicrobial prescribing behavior after the introduction of the antimicrobial stewardship program: A pre- and post-intervention survey. *Infect. Dis. Rep.* **2017**, *9*, 7268. [CrossRef]
14. Nault, V.; Pepin, J.; Beaudoin, M.; Perron, J.; Moutquin, J.M.; Valiquette, L. Sustained impact of a computer-assisted antimicrobial stewardship intervention on antimicrobial use and length of stay. *J. Antimicrob. Chemother.* **2017**, *72*, 933–940. [CrossRef]
15. Haseeb, A.; Faidah, H.S.; Al-Gethamy, M.; Iqbal, M.S.; Alhifany, A.A.; Ali, M.; Almarzoky Abuhussain, S.S.; Elrggal, M.E.; Almalki, W.H.; Alghamdi, S.; et al. Evaluation of Antimicrobial Stewardship Programs (ASPs) and their perceived level of success at Makkah region hospitals, Kingdom of Saudi Arabia. *Saudi Pharm. J.* **2020**, *28*, 1166–1171. [CrossRef]
16. Labricciosa, F.M.; Sartelli, M.; Correia, S.; Abbo, L.M.; Severo, M.; Ansaloni, L.; Coccolini, F.; Alves, C.; Melo, R.B.; Baiocchi, G.L.; et al. Emergency surgeons' perceptions and attitudes towards antibiotic prescribing and resistance: A worldwide cross-sectional survey. *World J. Emerg. Surg.* **2018**, *13*, 27. [CrossRef]
17. Charani, E.; Castro-Sanchez, E.; Holmes, A. The role of behavior change in antimicrobial stewardship. *Infect. Dis. Clin. N. Am.* **2014**, *28*, 169–175. [CrossRef]
18. Rizk, N.A.; Moghnieh, R.; Haddad, N.; Rebeiz, M.C.; Zeenny, R.M.; Hindy, J.R.; Orlando, G.; Kanj, S.S. Challenges to antimicrobial stewardship in the countries of the Arab League: Concerns of worsening resistance during the COVID-19 pandemic and proposed solutions. *Antibiotics (Basel)* **2021**, *10*, 1320. [CrossRef]

19. Mazdeyasna, H.; Nori, P.; Patel, P.; Doll, M.; Godbout, E.; Lee, K.; Noda, A.J.; Bearman, G.; Stevens, M.P. Antimicrobial stewardship at the core of COVID-19 response efforts: Implications for sustaining and building programs. *Curr. Infect. Dis. Rep.* **2020**, *22*, 23. [CrossRef]
20. van Limburg, M.; Sinha, B.; Lo-Ten-Foe, J.R.; van Gemert-Pijnen, J.E. Evaluation of early implementations of antibiotic stewardship program initiatives in nine Dutch hospitals. *Antimicrob. Resist. Infect. Control* **2014**, *3*, 33. [CrossRef]
21. Sayegh, N.; Hallit, S.; Hallit, R.; Saleh, N.; Zeidan, R.K. Physicians' attitudes on the implementation of an antimicrobial stewardship program in Lebanese hospitals. *Pharm. Pract. (Granada)* **2021**, *19*, 2192. [CrossRef]
22. Barlam, T.F.; Cosgrove, S.E.; Abbo, L.M.; MacDougall, C.; Schuetz, A.N.; Septimus, E.J.; Srinivasan, A.; Dellit, T.H.; Falck-Ytter, Y.T.; Fishman, N.O.; et al. Implementing an Antibiotic Stewardship Program: Guidelines by the Infectious Diseases Society of America and the Society for Healthcare Epidemiology of America. *Clin. Infect. Dis.* **2016**, *62*, e51–e77. [CrossRef]
23. Zhou, S.; Yang, Y.; Zhang, X.; Li, Z.; Liu, X.; Hu, C.; Chen, C.; Wang, D.; Peng, Z. Clinical course of 195 critically ill COVID-19 patients: A retrospective multicenter study. *Shock* **2020**, *54*, 644–651. [CrossRef]
24. Ruan, Q.; Yang, K.; Wang, W.; Jiang, L.; Song, J. Clinical predictors of mortality due to COVID-19 based on an analysis of data of 150 patients from Wuhan, China. *Intensive Care Med.* **2020**, *46*, 846–848. [CrossRef]
25. Hughes, S.; Troise, O.; Donaldson, H.; Mughal, N.; Moore, L.S.P. Bacterial and fungal coinfection among hospitalized patients with COVID-19: A retrospective cohort study in a UK secondary-care setting. *Clin. Microbiol. Infect.* **2020**, *26*, 1395–1399. [CrossRef]

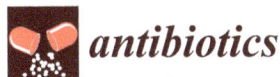

Article

Impact of Guideline Adherence on Outcomes in Patients Hospitalized with Community-Acquired Pneumonia (CAP) in Hungary: A Retrospective Observational Study

Adina Fésüs [1,2,3,4], Ria Benkő [5,6,7], Mária Matuz [5,6], Zsófia Engi [5], Roxána Ruzsa [5], Helga Hambalek [5], Árpád Illés [8] and Gábor Kardos [9,*]

1. Central Clinical Pharmacy, Clinical Center, University of Debrecen, H-4032 Debrecen, Hungary; fesus.adina@pharm.unideb.hu
2. Department of Pharmacodynamics, Faculty of Pharmacy, University of Debrecen, H-4032 Debrecen, Hungary
3. Doctoral School of Pharmaceutical Sciences, University of Debrecen, H-4032 Debrecen, Hungary
4. Health Industry Competence Centre, University of Debrecen, H-4032 Debrecen, Hungary
5. Clinical Pharmacy Department, Faculty of Pharmacy, University of Szeged, H-6725 Szeged, Hungary; benko.ria@med.u-szeged.hu (R.B.); matuz.maria@szte.hu (M.M.); engi.zsofia@szte.hu (Z.E.); roxana.ruzsa@gmail.com (R.R.); helgahambalek@gmail.com (H.H.)
6. Central Pharmacy, Albert Szent Györgyi Medical Center, University of Szeged, H-6725 Szeged, Hungary
7. Department of Emergency Medicine, Albert Szent Györgyi Medical Center, University of Szeged, H-6725 Szeged, Hungary
8. Department of Internal Medicine, Faculty of Medicine, University of Debrecen, H-4032 Debrecen, Hungary; illes.arpad@med.unideb.hu
9. Department of Metagenomics, University of Debrecen, H-4032 Debrecen, Hungary
* Correspondence: kg@med.unideb.hu

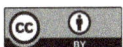

Citation: Fésüs, A.; Benkő, R.; Matuz, M.; Engi, Z.; Ruzsa, R.; Hambalek, H.; Illés, Á.; Kardos, G. Impact of Guideline Adherence on Outcomes in Patients Hospitalized with Community-Acquired Pneumonia (CAP) in Hungary: A Retrospective Observational Study. *Antibiotics* **2022**, *11*, 468. https://doi.org/10.3390/antibiotics11040468

Academic Editor: Masafumi Seki

Received: 25 February 2022
Accepted: 29 March 2022
Published: 30 March 2022

Publisher's Note: MDPI stays neutral with regard to jurisdictional claims in published maps and institutional affiliations.

Copyright: © 2022 by the authors. Licensee MDPI, Basel, Switzerland. This article is an open access article distributed under the terms and conditions of the Creative Commons Attribution (CC BY) license (https://creativecommons.org/licenses/by/4.0/).

Abstract: Community-acquired pneumonia (CAP) is a leading cause of morbidity and mortality worldwide. This retrospective observational study evaluated the antibiotic prescription patterns and associations between guideline adherence and outcomes in patients hospitalized with CAP in Hungary. Main outcome measures were adherence to national and international CAP guidelines (agent choice, dose) when using empirical antibiotics, antibiotic exposure, and clinical outcomes. Demographic and clinical characteristics of patients with CAP in the 30-day mortality and 30-day survival groups were compared. Fisher's exact test and t-test were applied to compare categorical and continuous variables, respectively. Adherence to the national CAP guideline for initial empirical therapies was 30.61% (45/147) for agent choice and 88.89% (40/45) for dose. Average duration of antibiotic therapy for CAP was 7.13 ± 4.37 (mean ± SD) days, while average antibiotic consumption was 11.41 ± 8.59 DDD/patient (range 1–44.5). Adherence to national guideline led to a slightly lower 30-day mortality rate than guideline non-adherence (15.56% vs. 16.67%, $p > 0.05$). In patients aged ≥ 85 years, 30-day mortality was 3 times higher than in those aged 65–84 years (30.43% vs. 11.11%). A significant difference was found between 30-day non-survivors and 30-day survivors regarding the average CRP values on admission (177.28 ± 118.94 vs. 112.88 ± 93.47 mg/L, respectively, $p = 0.006$) and CCI score (5.71 ± 1.85 and 4.67 ± 1.83, $p = 0.012$). We found poor adherence to the national and international CAP guidelines in terms of agent choice. In addition, high CRP values on admission were markedly associated with higher mortality in CAP.

Keywords: community acquired pneumonia; hospitalized patients; empirical antibiotic therapy; guideline adherence; clinical outcomes; 30-day mortality; CRP on admission; CCI score

1. Introduction

The use of antibiotics has significantly reduced bacterial infection-related morbidity and mortality; their inappropriate use, however, has led to the emergence of antibiotic resistance at the same time [1,2].

The epicenter of antibiotic resistance is the hospital environment; thus, it is critical to rationalize antibiotic use in this setting. In European acute-care hospitals, 35% of patients receive systemic antibiotics during their stay [3]. European Centre for Disease Prevention and Control (ECDC) point prevalence survey data showed that antibiotic use for community acquired infections (CAIs) in Europe represented 69.9% of all antibacterial use in acute-care hospitals [4]. In particular, more than one-third (35%) of CAIs were found to be respiratory tract infections (RTIs) [5]. In 2016, respiratory illnesses were the third most common cause of death in Europe, and accounted for 7.5% of all deaths, while in 2017 the corresponding number in Hungary was 6.2% [6]. Community-acquired pneumonia (CAP) is one of the most common and potentially serious infectious diseases and is still one of the leading causes of morbidity and mortality worldwide [7–9], imposing a heavy economic burden on health systems even in developed countries. In European countries, CAP was responsible for almost 30% of mortality in the category of respiratory illnesses in 2015 [10]. Although CAP is often treated in ambulatory settings, hospitalization rates range from 30% to 60% [11]. Recent CDC data found that in the United States, 79% of all patients with CAP were treated inappropriately in the hospital setting [12]. Inappropriateness of hospital treatment of CAP is associated with worse therapy outcomes, longer hospital stays, and higher cost of treatment [13–17]. The National Institute for Health and Care Excellence and British Thoracic Society (NICE/BTS) and the American Thoracic Society and the Infectious Diseases Society of America (ATS/IDSA) have published official clinical CAP guidelines making recommendations for selection of initial empiric antibiotic therapy for patients hospitalized with CAP. A national CAP guideline has also been published by the Hungarian Professional Society of Infectious Diseases and Pulmonology.

To date, descriptions of antibiotic treatment trends for CAP have only been published for adult outpatient care in Hungary [18]. Despite the importance and incidence of CAP, no field studies have been performed in Hungarian hospitals to assess the initiated antibiotic treatments.

The aim of this study was to evaluate the characteristics and outcome of antibacterial drug use in patients admitted to hospital due to CAP. The primary aims were to evaluate adherence to national and international antibacterial guidelines and to analyze the potential factors associated with mortality. Secondly, we reported some basic characteristics of antibacterial treatments used in CAP.

2. Results

In the study period, data of 1665 patients were collected, out of which data obtained from 147 patients met the study criteria and could be included in the analysis.

2.1. Patient Characteristics and Main Outcomes

The characteristics of patients and their comorbidities are described in Table 1. A total of 64 (43.54%) male patients hospitalized due to CAP were included in the study. Their age at hospital admission ranged from 27 to 95 years; 118 (80.27%) patients were aged ≥ 65 years (Table 1). Overall, 59.86% of patients had a CCI score above 4. The most common comorbidities included cardiovascular diseases (35.37%) and diabetes mellitus (22.45%) (Table 1). The majority of patients were discharged home (80.95%), and only a small proportion were admitted to ICU (7.48%). The overall 30-day mortality rate was 24 (16.33%) (Table 1), comprising 15 (62.5%) in-hospital deaths and 9 (37.5%) post-discharge deaths.

Table 1. Demographic and clinical characteristics of patients with CAP.

Parameter	N	%
	147	100
Gender (Male)	64	43.54
Age		
20–64 years	29	19.73
65–84 years	72	48.98
≥85 years	46	31.29
Penicillin allergy	2	1.36
CCI—Charlson comorbidity index		
0	3	2.04
1	2	1.36
2	10	6.80
3	12	8.16
4	32	21.77
>4	88	59.86
Comorbidities		
Cardiovascular disease	52	35.37
Diabetes mellitus	33	22.45
Chronic obstructive pulmonary disease	13	8.84
Chronic liver/kidney disease (moderate to severe)	11	7.48
Hematologic malignant diseases	8	5.44
Solid tumor		
Localized	2	1.36
Metastatic	6	4.08
Peripheral vascular disease	5	3.40
Dementia	3	2.04
Peptic ulcer disease	2	1.36
Cerebrovascular accident or transient ischemic attack	1	0.68
Discharge types		
Discharged home	119	80.95
Moved to another hospital ward	2	1.36
Intensive care unit (ICU)	11	7.48
Outcome		
In-hospital mortality	15	10.20
30-day mortality	24	16.33
Length of stay (LOS) (mean ± SD)-days	8.26 ± 5.64 (1–33) *	

SD—standard deviation; * Data are presented as mean ± standard deviation (min–max).

2.2. Guideline Adherence

Amoxicillin–clavulanic acid was the most widely used antibiotic therapy, administered to 29.07% of patients in monotherapy and 54.09% of patients in combination, followed by ceftriaxone (monotherapy: 29.07%, combination: 25.59%) and moxifloxacin (monotherapy: 19.77%, combination: 16.39%) (Table 2). Guideline adherence (agent choice) rates to national, BTS/NICE, and ATS/IDSA CAP guidelines are presented in Table 3. Initial empirical therapies for CAP showed a relatively low rate of guideline adherence: 30.61% for national, 22.45% for BTS/NICE, and 15.65% for ATS/IDSA CAP guidelines. The rate of adherence to at least one guideline was 34.69% (Table 3).

Table 2. The distribution of first empirical antibiotic therapies (mono- and combination therapies).

Antibiotics	Frequency (N)	%	Guideline Adherence		
			National	BTS/NICE/NICE	ATS/IDSA
Monotherapies (N = 86; 100%)					
Amoxicillin-clavulanic acid	25	29.07			
Ceftriaxone	25	29.07			
Moxifloxacin	17	19.77	✓		✓
Levofloxacin	6	6.98	✓	✓	✓
Clarithromycin	5	5.81		✓	
Meropenem	4	4.65			
Amoxicillin	1	1.16		✓	
Doxycycline	1	1.16		✓	
Metronidazole	1	1.16			
Norfloxacin	1	1.16			
Combination therapies (N = 61; 100%)					
amoxicillin-clavulanic acid + clarithromycin	23	37.70	✓	✓	
moxifloxacin + metronidazole	7	11.48			
ceftriaxone + metronidazole	6	9.84			
amoxicillin-clavulanic acid + metronidazole	5	8.20			
amoxicillin-clavulanic acid + clarithromycin + metronidazole	3	4.92			
ceftriaxone + clarithromycin	2	3.28	✓		✓
ceftriaxone + metronidazole + clarithromycin	2	3.28			
ceftriaxone + sulphamethoxazole and trimethoprim	2	3.28			
amoxicillin-clavulanic acid + clarithromycin + amikacin	1	1.64			
amoxicillin-clavulanic acid + flucloxacillin	1	1.64			
ceftriaxone + metronidazole + sulphamethoxazole and trimethoprim	1	1.64			
ceftriaxone + moxifloxacin	1	1.64			✓
levofloxacin + metronidazole	1	1.64			
meropenem + metronidazole	1	1.64			
moxifloxacin + flucloxacillin	1	1.64			
moxifloxacin + metronidazole + ceftriaxone	1	1.64			
piperacillin/tazobactame + amikacin	1	1.64			
piperacillin/tazobactame + metronidazole	1	1.64			
meropenem + vancomycin	1	1.64			

ATS/IDSA—American Thoracic Society/Infectious Diseases Society of America; BTS/NICE—British Thoracic Society/National Institute for Health and Care Excellence; ✓—guideline adherence.

Table 3. Characteristics of antibiotic therapies.

Parameters	N	%
	147	100
Adherence to the national guideline (agent choice)	45	30.61
Adherence to BTS/NICE guideline (agent choice)	33	22.45
Adherence to ATS/IDSA guideline (agent choice)	23	15.65
Adherence to at least one guideline (agent choice)	51	34.69
Type of the first antibiotic therapy		
Combination therapies	61	41.50
Monotherapies	86	58.50
Most common therapies		
beta-lactams and macrolide	25	17.01
beta-lactams	51	34.69
respiratory fluoroquinolones	23	15.65
Route of administration of the first antibiotic therapy		
iv	93	63.27
oral	54	36.73
Duration of total antibiotic therapies		
short therapy (1–6 days)	120	81.63
long therapy ($\geq$ 7 days)	27	18.37
Number of consecutive antibiotic therapies		
1	85	57.8
>1 (2–4)	62	42.2
Changes in the first empirical therapy		
Sequential antibiotic therapy*	14	9.52
De-escalation	6	4.08
Escalation	42	28.57
No change	85	57.8

BTS/NICE—British Thoracic Society/National Institute for Health and Care Excellence; ATS/IDSA—American Thoracic Society/Infectious Diseases Society of America; iv—intravenously; * switch from an IV to oral regimen.

Dosage appropriateness assessments are shown in Table 4. In line with the previous section, the highest guideline adherence (agent, dose) rate was found in relation to the national guideline (40/45, 88.89%), followed by ATS/IDSA (18/23, 78.26%) and BTS/NICE (24/33, 72.73%) CAP guidelines.

2.3. Antibiotic Therapy for CAP

The characteristics of first antibiotic therapies and key outcomes are described in Table 3. The majority of treatments (58.50%) were monotherapies; 93 (63.27%) patients received the first antibacterial therapy IV (intravenously), and 14 of them (15.05%) were switched to oral route within 1–5 (median 3.5) days.

The average duration of antibiotic therapy for CAP was 7.13 ± 4.37 days (median 6, range 1–27), while the average antibiotic consumption was 11.41 ± 8.59 DDD/patient (range 1–44.5). The majority of patients (81.63%) received short-term (1–6 days) antibiotic therapy. In the majority of cases, there was no change in the first empirical therapy (85/147, 57.8%). However, changes occurred due to sequential antibiotic therapy (9.52%), de-escalation (4.08%), and escalation (28.57%) (Table 3). A significant difference was found in the 30-day mortality rate between these types of antibiotic therapies (no change: 12.94%, sequential antibiotic therapy: 0%, de-escalation: 0%, and escalation: 30.95%, $p = 0.046$).

Table 4. Guideline adherence, N = 147 patients.

	Adherence Frequency	%
AB1-National CAP guideline adherence	45	100
appropriate use	40	88.89
overdose (compared to SPC, due to lack of guideline recommended dose)	4	8.89
underdose (due to body weight)	1	2.22
AB1-BTS/NICE CAP guideline adherence	33	100
appropriate use	24	72.73
underdose (compared to guideline)	4	12.12
overdose (in case of low levels of eGFR)	4	12.12
debatable use (absence of loading dose)	1	3.03
AB1-ATS/IDSA CAP guideline adherence	23	100
appropriate use	18	78.26
underdose (compared to guideline)	3	13.04
overdose (in case of low levels of eGFR)	2	8.70

AB1—first empirical antibiotic treatment; CAP—community acquired pneumonia; SPC—summary of product characteristics; BTS/NICE—British Thoracic Society/National Institute for Health and Care Excellence; eGFR—estimated glomerular filtration rate; ATS/IDSA—American Thoracic Society/Infectious Diseases Society of America.

2.4. Clinical Outcomes: LOS, 30-Day Mortality

In our study, the mean LOS was 8.26 ± 5.64 (range 1–33) days (Table 1). Adherence to the national guideline led to a slightly lower 30-day mortality rate than guideline non-adherence (15.56% vs. 16.67%, $p > 0.05$), while this difference was more pronounced in the case of international guidelines (BTS/NICE: 21.21% vs. 14.91%, and ATS/IDSA: 21.74 vs. 15.32%, $p > 0.05$) (Table 3). Furthermore, we found that the 30-day mortality rate for the different types of therapies was as follows: 8% for combination of beta-lactam and macrolide, 19.61% for beta-lactam monotherapies, and 21.77% for respiratory fluoroquinolone monotherapies ($p > 0.05$).

2.5. Prognostic Factors for Mortality in CAP

The demographic and clinical characteristics of 30-day survivors (123/147, 83.67%) and non-survivors are compared in Table 5.

We observed a significant difference in the 30-day mortality of CAP between age groups. The 30-day mortality rate increased proportionally with age: it was 6.90% (2/29) among patients aged 20–64 years, 11.11% (8/72) in patients aged 65–84 years, and reached 30.43% (14/46) in the 85+ age group (Table 5).

The CCI score of patients in the 30-day non-survivor group was higher by one point on average (5.71 ± 1.85 vs. 4.67 ± 1.83, $p = 0.012$) (Table 5).

In terms of C-reactive protein (CRP) levels at admission, a remarkable difference was found between the two patient groups (30-day non-survivor: 177.28 ± 118.94 vs. 30-day survivor: 112.88 ± 93.47 mg/L, $p = 0.006$) (Table 5).

Thirty-day mortality was not associated with significantly longer LOS (9.54 ± 8.45 vs. 8.01 ± 4.93 days, $p = 0.668$), higher antibiotic exposure (8.25 vs. 7.98 DDD/patient, $p = 0.21$), or longer duration of antibiotic therapy (8.20 ± 7.03 vs. 6.92 ± 3.64 days, $p = 0.187$). Similarly, we found a median 1-day difference between 30-day survivors and non-survivors in the duration of antibiotic therapies (6 vs. 7 days, respectively), and length of stay (7 vs. 8 days, respectively).

Table 5. Comparison of baseline and clinical characteristics of 30-day non-survivors and survivors among patients with CAP.

		30-Day Survival		
		Non-Survivors	Survivors	p-Value
Total		24 (16.33%)	123 (83.67%)	-
Gender	male	9 (14.06%)	55 (85.94%)	0.654
	female	15 (18.07%)	68 (81.93%)	
Age (years)	mean ± SD	81.57 ± 10.77	75.12 ± 13.43	0.028
	20–64	2 (6.90%)	27 (93.1%)	-
	65–84	8 (11.11%)	64 (88.89%)	
	85+	14 (30.43%)	32 (69.57%)	
CCI score	mean ± SD	5.71 ± 1.85	4.67 ± 1.83	0.012
Diabetes mellitus	yes	7 (21.21%)	26 (78.79%)	0.425
	no	17 (14.91%)	97 (85.09%)	
Leukemia	yes	5 (13.89%)	31 (86.11%)	0.798
	no	19 (17.12%)	92 (82.88%)	
Chronic kidney disease	yes	4 (57.14%)	3 (42.86%)	0.014
	no	20 (14.29%)	120 (85.71%)	
Congestive heart failure	yes	6 (12.77%)	41 (87.23%)	0.482
	no	18 (18%)	82 (82%)	
Type of therapy	combination	6 (9.84%)	55 (90.16%)	0.112
	monotherapy	18 (20.93%)	68 (79.07%)	
National CAP guideline adherence	adherent	7 (15.56%)	38 (84.44%)	1.000
	non-adherent	17 (16.67%)	85 (83.33%)	
BTS/NICE CAP guideline adherence	adherent	7 (21.21%)	26 (78.79%)	0.425
	non-adherent	17 (14.91%)	97 (85.09%)	
ATS/IDSA CAP guideline adherence	adherent	5 (21.74%)	18 (78.26%)	0.538
	non-adherent	19 (15.32%)	105 (84.68%)	
CRP (mg/L) at admission	mean ± SD	177.28 ± 118.94	112.88 ± 93.47	0.006
	high levels (8<)	20 (16.67%)	101 (83.47%)	0.449
	normal levels (0–8)	1 (8.33%)	10 (90.91%)	
	NA	3 (20%)	12 (80%)	-

SD—standard deviation; CCI—Charlson comorbidity index; CAP—community acquired pneumonia; BTS/NICE—British Thoracic Society/National Institute for Health and Care Excellence; ATS/IDSA—American Thoracic Society/Infectious Diseases Society of America; CRP—C-reactive protein; NA—not available. p-value: Fisher's exact test was performed for categorical variables, and t-test was used to compare continuous variables between groups.

The results of logistic regression analysis are displayed in Table 6. Out of the three factors (increased age, higher CCI score, and higher CRP level) that were associated with higher mortality in the univariate analysis, only the CRP level on admission was found to increase the risk of mortality. Each additional increase of 50 mg/L in the CRP level seen on admission increased the 30-day mortality odds 1.3-fold, indicating that the degree of inflammation affects mortality.

Table 6. CCI scores and CRP levels on admission in non-surviving and surviving patients' groups with odds ratio.

	B	S.E.	p-Value	OR	95% CI for OR	
					Lower	Upper
Age (years)	0.058	0.032	0.072	1.059	0.995	1.128
CCI score	0.203	0.155	0.191	1.2259	0.904	1.659
CRP 9 category *	0.289	0.125	0.020	1.3362	1.046	1.705
Constant	−8.562	2.675	0.001	0.000		

B—regression coefficient; S.E.—standard error; OR—odds ratio; CI—confidence interval; CCI—Charlson comorbidity index; CRP—C-reactive protein; * CRP 9 categories: 1: 0–8 (mg/L); 2: 8–50 (mg/L); 3: 50–100 (mg/L); 4: 100–150 (mg/L); 5: 150–200 (mg/L); 6: 200–250 (mg/L); 7: 250–300 (mg/L); 8: 300–350 (mg/L); 9: above 350 (mg/L).

3. Discussion

Even though CAP is one of the most common acute infections, ours is the first field study in Hungary that has been conducted regarding the evaluation of antibiotic prescription patterns, associations between guideline adherence and outcomes in patients with CAP who required hospitalization.

3.1. CAP Guidelines

Based on ATS/IDSA and BTS/NICE CAP guidelines, combinations of beta-lactams and macrolides, or respiratory fluoroquinolones (RFQs) are recommended as first choice agents to treat empirically moderate-severe (hospitalized in non-ICU ward) CAP [19,20].

The Hungarian guideline for patients hospitalized with CAP is similar to international guidelines in terms of agent selection [21]. This guideline recommends the use of respiratory fluoroquinolones (moxifloxacin or levofloxacin) as monotherapy or the combination of beta-lactam (amoxicillin clavulanic acid or ceftriaxone) and clarithromycin to cover both typical (e.g., *Streptococcus pneumoniae*, *Haemophilus influenzae*, *Staphylococcus aureus*, Group A streptococci, *Moraxella catarrhalis*) and atypical pathogens (e.g., *Legionella*, *Mycoplasma pneumoniae*, *Chlamydia pneumoniae*) responsible for CAP.

3.1.1. Guideline Adherence: Agent Selection

Among the patients hospitalized with CAP investigated in the present study, the rate of national guideline adherence for antibiotic selection was 30.61% (N = 45). The most common guideline adherent empirical treatment for CAP was amoxicillin-clavulanic acid combined with clarithromycin, or moxifloxacin or levofloxacin as monotherapy (23, 47.92% in both cases), followed by ceftriaxone combined with clarithromycin (2, 4.16%). In 2017, national surveillance data for antibiotic resistance in hospitalized patients still reported relatively high susceptibility rates for the antibacterial agents used against *S. pneumonia* (98.5% to ceftriaxone, 96.3% to levofloxacin, 96.2% to moxifloxacin 93.8% to ampicillin, and 74.7% to macrolides). Additionally, amoxicillin clavulanic acid showed potent activity (94.4%) against *H. influenza* strains [22].

Guideline adherent empirical antibiotic use in CAP is quite varied in the related literature. Three studies evaluating patients hospitalized with CAP found guideline adherent antibiotic therapy in 57%, 57%, and 65% of the cases [16,17,23]; these rates were higher compared to our results. At the same time, an Italian multicenter before-and-after guideline implementation survey found that guideline adherent antibiotic prescribing increased significantly (33 vs. 44 %; $p < 0.001$) [24] compared to a poor initial guideline adherence, similar to our results. The low guideline adherence found in our study may be explained by the fact that although there was a Hungarian guideline, its dissemination and accessibility were not adequate; consequently, it had not been integrated in daily practice.

3.1.2. Guideline Adherence: Dosing

Even though we found high adherence to the national guideline in terms of dosing (88.89%), over- and underdosing still affected relatively high proportions of patients (8.89% and 2.22%, respectively). Overdosing occurred most commonly in renal impairment, when dose adjustment would have been required for amoxicillin-clavulanic acid, clarithromycin, and moxifloxacin. The other common error occurred mostly due to routine underdosing of levofloxacin and clarithromycin, or not taking into account patients' extreme body weights (Appendix A: Table A1).

3.2. Changes in the First Empirical Therapy

Considering the route of administration, the majority of patients (63.27%) received IV initial antibacterial therapy for CAP. At the same time, switching from an IV to oral regimen (in 9.52% of the cases) was performed within 1–5 (median 3.5) days. These results are mostly supported by the national and international guidelines, according to which the empirical antibiotic treatment in patients hospitalized with CAP can be initiated via any route, but using antibiotics exclusively intravenously is only recommended when the oral route is compromised. The review of intravenous antibiotics after 48 h of use and switching to oral antibiotics are recommended, if possible, when either the same agent or the same drug class should be used [19,20]. According to the ATS/IDSA guideline, patients hospitalized with CAP should be switched from intravenous to oral therapy when they are hemodynamically stable, showing signs of clinical improvement (within the first 48–72 h), are able to ingest medications, and have a normally functioning gastrointestinal tract [25]. At the same time, according to a multicenter randomized clinical trial performed in four teaching hospitals in Spain, the switch from intravenous to oral regimen is not currently common in clinical practice [26].

In addition, more antibiotic therapy needed further escalation (28.57%), while changes in the first empirical therapy due to de-escalation (4.08%) occurred at relatively low rates.

The guidelines for CAP stress the importance of de-escalation of empirical antibiotic therapy, recommending the stricter use of broad-spectrum antibiotics [19,20]. Although appropriate dosage and de-escalation are important in optimizing antibiotic use and reducing antibiotic resistance, studies dealing with antibiotic dosing in CAP treatments are rare. A cross-sectional study in Australian patients hospitalized with CAP found that the most common errors in high-risk CAP were inappropriate dose, route, and duration, which affected 69% (N = 27) of patients. Routine underdosing of ceftriaxone was the most frequent (N = 17, 44%), while 54% of patients were prescribed antibiotics to administer via a route not recommended on the basis of CAP severity [27]. According to a multicenter study in the Netherlands, where de-escalation occurred in 16.7% of the patients hospitalized with CAP, physicians seem to be more inclined to continue the regimen when it appears to be effective [28].

3.3. Duration of Antibiotic Therapy

Our results are in line with the requirements of international guidelines [19,20]: most of our patients (81.63%) receive short antibiotic therapy (1–6 days), while the median duration of antibiotic therapies for CAP was 6 days (range 1–27).

The optimal duration of antimicrobial therapy in CAP is not well-established. Although the national CAP guideline for in-patients does not cover the duration of antibiotic treatment, according to the ATS/IDSA guideline, patients hospitalized with CAP should be treated for a minimum of 5 days [25]. Additionally, in inpatient settings, a small number of studies have addressed the appropriate duration of antibiotic therapy in CAP. A recent meta-analysis of patients hospitalized with CAP demonstrated the efficacy of shorter courses of antibiotic therapy (of 5 to 7 days) [29]. Despite recommendations, a recent international audit found that prolonged antibiotic therapy for CAP was common and frequently observed due to the presence of comorbidities [30].

3.4. Clinical Outcomes: 30-Day Mortality

Regarding clinical outcomes, in the present study we found that guideline adherence to national recommendations was associated with slightly lower 30-day mortality than guideline non-adherence (15.56% vs. 16.67%, $p > 0.05$). Furthermore, studies showed that both in Europe and the United States, guideline adherence in patients hospitalized with CAP was associated with lower 30-day mortality [13–15]. Nevertheless, another multicenter cross-sectional study reported that no significant difference was found between guideline adherent and non-adherent antibiotic prescribing episodes and inpatient mortality (1.6% vs. 4.1%; $p = 0.18$) [31].

Several studies have focused on the relation between mono- or combination therapies and clinical outcomes [32,33]. The results of a multicenter study in patients admitted to non-ICU wards with CAP have shown clinical outcomes, recovery rate and mortality to be unaffected by the choice of a beta-lactam, beta-lactam and macrolide, or respiratory fluoroquinolone antibiotic regimen [32]. According to a systematic review on antibiotic therapy for non-ICU hospitalized patients with CAP, fluoroquinolone monotherapy had similar efficacy and favorable safety compared to beta-lactam with or without macrolide [34]; however, the authors pointed out several quality issues and recommended further good quality research to confirm these findings [34].

In the present study, we found a slightly better mortality rate in CAP hospitalized patients with the combination of beta-lactam and macrolide, compared with beta-lactam or respiratory fluoroquinolone monotherapies (8% vs. 19.61% and 21.77%, respectively, $p > 0.05$).

Further, changes in the first empirical therapy due to de-escalation (4.08%) and switching from intravenous to oral regimen (9.52%) occurred relatively infrequently, and were not associated with increased 30-day mortality rates (0% for both). Admittedly, we conducted the survey on a relatively small number of cases. A simulation study embedded in a prospective cohort (performed in 58 hospitals) found that 30-day mortality in patients hospitalized with CAP was 3.5% and 10.9% in the de-escalation and continuation groups, respectively. At the same time, the simulation study also suggested that the effect of de-escalation on mortality needs further evaluation to determine effect size more accurately [28].

Regarding the duration of antibiotic therapy, we found no difference in mortality rates between short- and long-term therapies (16.67% vs. 14.81%, $p > 0.05$), which may suggest that short antibiotic therapy can be as effective as long antibiotic therapy. A previous meta-analysis of five randomized trials (which included patients of all ages, excluded neonates, and any severity of CAP) found no differences in clinical outcome and mortality rates comparing short (1–6 days) versus long (≥ 7 days) antibacterial therapies [35]. Our results support these finding by showing similar mortality rates for both short and long antibiotic durations.

3.5. Prognostic Factors for Mortality Due to CAP

Previous research found that increased age, male gender, increased CRP, and comorbid conditions (mainly malignancy, congestive heart failure, diabetes mellitus, and renal disease) act as predictive factors for mortality in patients hospitalized with CAP [36–38].

As for age, our results show that 30-day mortality in patients aged ≥ 85 years was 3-fold compared with those aged 65–84 years (30.43% vs. 11.11%). Studies found that age ≥ 85 years was an independent predictive factor for mortality in CAP, increasing the risk of death significantly [36,37]. According to Torner et al., age ≥ 85 years was markedly associated with mortality in CAP, since the 30-day mortality rate was 2.6 times higher in this age group compared with patients aged between 65 and 84 years [39]. Moreover, Luna et al. concluded that an age of 80 years or more should already be considered a risk factor for poor outcome in CAP [40].

Furthermore, a temporal analysis of pneumonia (excluding influenza-related pneumonia, aspirational pneumonia, and congenital pneumonia) mortality rates in European countries between 2001 and 2014 revealed gender discrepancy: mortality was higher in males than in females [41]. Regarding Hungary, a mortality rate of 7.46% in males and 3.72% in females was reported [41]. Surprisingly, the mortality rate in the present study was higher among females than males (18.07 vs. 14.06%). However, this difference is not clinically significant. Even though in the study population there were more females (56.46%) than males, we cannot give an obvious explanation for these mortality rates, since CCI and CRP did not differ across genders.

The other commonly studied prognostic factor for CAP mortality is CRP level. The CRP test is the most widely used serum biomarker in the differential diagnosis (viral or bacterial etiology) of lower respiratory tract infections. Due to bacterial infection, CRP levels rise within the first 6 to 8 h in response to several inflammatory stimuli.

Several studies evaluated the relationship between C-reactive protein serum level and outcomes of CAP. Mendez et al. and Summah et al. concluded that CRP values increase in line with the severity of CAP, and can be used as an independent prognostic predictor of the severity of CAP, for the follow-up of patients' condition, for response to antibiotic therapy, and CAP clinical outcome [42–45]. Moreover, CRP level may guide CAP empirical treatment decisions and help avoid unnecessary antibiotic use in hospitalized patients [46,47]. A recent study conducted in a Scottish hospital demonstrated that a CRP level below 100 mg/L on admission was significantly associated with reduced 30-day mortality (OR 0.18, p = 0.03) [48]. In a Danish teaching hospital, the highest mortality risk was found in patients with CRP > 75 mg/L on admission [49]. Results of the present study are consistent with these previous findings, as we recorded significantly higher average CRP values on admission in the group of patients who died within 30 days compared to 30-day survivors (177.28 ± 118.94 vs. 112.88 ± 93.47 mg/L, p = 0.006).

Regarding comorbid conditions, we found that CCI scores differed significantly between the 30-day non-surviving and 30-day surviving patients (5.71 ± 1.85 and 4.67 ± 1.83, p = 0.012). A higher CCI score due to the presence of comorbidities was associated with higher mortality rates (CCI score 0–4: 11.86%, CCI score 5–10: 19.32%) in CAP, similar to other literature data. A secondary analysis of CAP performed by Luna et al. found that the presence of comorbidities was associated with poorer outcomes [40].

3.6. Strengths and Limitations

The collected data provide detailed, first-hand observations on the everyday use of antibiotics in the empirical treatment of CAP in internal medicine hospitals. However, retrospective data collection from medical records might contain inaccuracies and potential biases.

One of the most important limitations of this study was that no clinical case definition of CAP was given or standardized at hospital level. However, the diagnosis of pneumonia was confirmed in every case by chest radiography. The second limitation was the lack of knowledge of pneumonia severity score (PSI score), since not all elements of the score were retrievable from medical records. Furthermore, there were no set hospital standard guidelines for the empirical antibiotic treatment of CAP. Therefore, national and international guidelines were used for assessing antibiotic use. Third, we also consider it likely that de-escalation (prescribing an oral antibiotic) occurred after discharge. However, no data were collected on de-escalation after discharge.

In conclusion, this study provides further evidence that guideline adherence in choosing the empirical antibiotic improves survival, and thus contributes to improvement of acceptance of antimicrobial stewardship. The results also draw attention to the need for improvement of empirical prescribing by limiting unnecessary combinations and by optimizing doses, especially in the cases of patients with higher CRP, In our country, there are few studies that explore those important healthcare practices at the individual patient level that may lead to the development of antimicrobial resistance. We believe that our results may contribute to optimizing CAP treatment in the future.

4. Materials and Methods

4.1. Study Design and Setting

A 1-year (January–December 2017) retrospective observational study was conducted at the 110-bed internal medicine unit of the University of Debrecen, which is a tertiary care teaching hospital.

4.2. Data Collection

Data for all inpatients receiving antibacterial therapy during the hospital stay were recorded by the ward pharmacist. All patient and therapy related data were collected manually from medication charts and discharge letters using the e-MedSolution Hospital Information System. Data collection forms were developed and the following data were extracted: patient age, sex, weight, date of hospital admission and discharge, comorbidities, discharge type. Clinical outcome (30-day mortality) and laboratory test results on the day of admission (white blood cell count, CRP, eGFR—estimated glomerular filtration rate) were also collected. In relation to the antibacterial therapy, the following data were collected: pre-hospital antibiotic therapy, drug allergy, indication of antibiotic treatment, empirical antibiotic choice, dosage, route of administration, and duration of antibacterial therapy during hospital stay. The extracted data were entered into Microsoft Excel spreadsheets for further analysis.

Only adult (18 years or above) patients who started their first empirical antibacterial therapy for community acquired pneumonia were included in the study. Empirical treatment was defined as antibacterial therapy without pathogen identification and susceptibility testing. Inclusion and exclusion criteria for the study are shown in Figure 1.

Patients' general condition was evaluated using the Charlson comorbidity index (CCI) [50]. eGFR on admission was used to assess dose appropriateness for drugs excreted renally. To reveal the antibiotic exposure of patients, the World Health Organization's ATC/DDD index (version 2021) was applied. Defined daily dose (DDD) refers to the assumed average maintenance dose per day for a drug used for its main indication in adults. Regarding antibiotics, DDD refers to infections of moderate severity [51]. Our analysis focused on systemic antibacterial drugs (ATC: J01). LOS refers to the number of days that patients spent in hospital. Both the admission and discharge day were counted as a separate day.

4.3. Main Outcome Measures

The primary outcome measure was guideline adherence to the national (published by Hungarian Professional College of Infectious Diseases and Pulmonology) and two international (ATS/IDSA-American Thoracic Society/Infectious Diseases Society of America, BTS/NICE-British Thoracic Society/National Institute for Health *and* Care Excellence) CAP guidelines, in terms of choice of empirical antibiotic(s) and dosing. Therefore, empirical treatment was considered guideline adherent when complying with the recommendations.

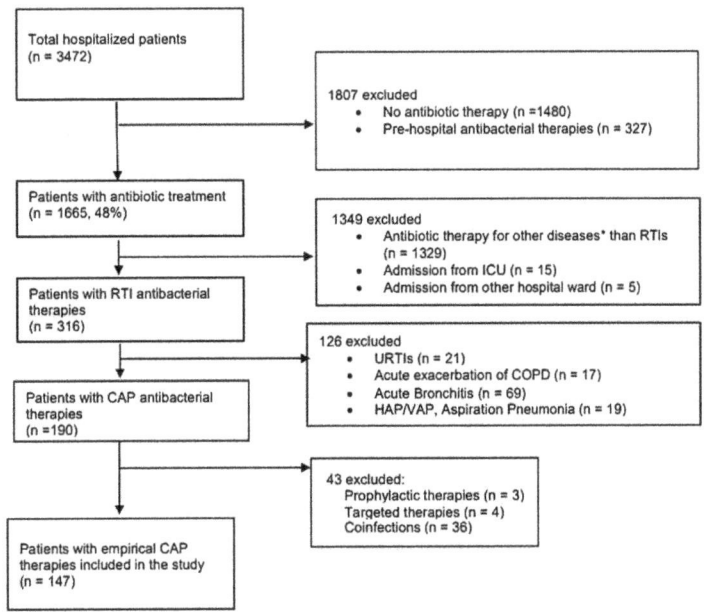

Figure 1. Flowchart for exclusion and inclusion criteria. * Other diseases: e.g., sepsis, urinary tract infection, etc.; RTIs—respiratory tract infections; ICU—intensive care unit; URTIs—upper respiratory tract infections; COPD—chronic obstructive pulmonary diseases; HAP—hospital acquired pneumonia; VAP—ventilation associated pneumonia; CAP—community acquired pneumonia.

Secondary outcome measures included antibiotic exposure (DDD/patient), and clinical outcome (30-day mortality rate).

Furthermore, demographic (age, gender) and clinical characteristics (CCI, CRP) of patients with CAP in the 30-day mortality and 30-day survivor groups were compared.

Assessment for guideline adherence was performed separately for each guideline as follows:

Choice assessment: The first empiric antibiotic therapy initiated for patients hospitalized with CAP was matched with guideline recommendations on antibiotic choice, and classified as adherent or non-adherent. Combined therapy was considered guideline adherent when all antibacterial agents of the combination were adherent. Non-immunocompetent patients (malignancy) were excluded from guideline adherence analysis, as the guidelines did not cover this special population.

Dosage assessment: The dose of the first guideline adherent empiric antibiotic therapy was established on the basis of the guidelines mentioned above, and defined as follows:

- *appropriate dose:* dose recommended by guidelines, administration of loading dose when recommended, and dose adjustment in renal impairment.
- *debatable dose:* under- or overdose by <50% compared to the dose recommended by guidelines, and/or absence of loading dose.
- *under-or overdose:* under- or overdose by ≥50% compared to the dose recommended by guidelines, and/or no dose adjustment in renal impairment and in extremes for body weight.

In cases of extreme body weight (<40 and >100 kg) and impaired renal function, the summary of product characteristics (SPC) was also considered, as it gives a detailed description about how to take into account body weight and eGFR in dose calculation. Dosing assessment was not performed for therapies considered as non-adherent regarding the antibiotic choice.

Changes in the first antibacterial treatment (sequential therapy: switch from an IV to oral regimen, de-escalation or escalation) were also assessed. Narrowing spectrum was considered de-escalation, while adding a new antibiotic or switching to a broader-spectrum agent was defined as escalation of the antibiotic regimen.

Clinical outcome assessment: The clinical outcome assessment was performed to see whether adherence to CAP guidelines improved 30-day mortality, and to map the predictive factors for mortality in patients hospitalized with CAP.

4.4. Statistical Analyses

Quantile–quantile plots (Q–Q plots) and density plots were used for checking normality of data visually. Fisher's exact test was applied to compare categorical variables, and t-test was used to compare continuous variables between groups. Significant p values were defined as below 0.05.

Patients were anonymized, thus made unidentifiable in the study.

5. Conclusions

We found poor adherence to the national and international CAP guidelines in terms of agent choice. In addition, CRP value on admission was markedly associated with mortality in CAP.

Author Contributions: Conceptualization, A.F., R.B., G.K. and M.M.; methodology, A.F., M.M., H.H., R.B., R.R. and Z.E.; validation M.M., Z.E., Á.I. and R.B.; formal analysis, A.F., H.H., R.R., G.K. and M.M.; investigation, A.F., R.R, Z.E. and R.B.; resources, Á.I. and G.K.; data curation, A.F.; writing—original draft preparation, A.F., Z.E, H.H., R.R. and R.B.; writing—review and editing, A.F., R.B., M.M. and G.K.; visualization, A.F. and M.M.; supervision, Á.I. and G.K. All authors have read and agreed to the published version of the manuscript.

Funding: This research received no external funding.

Institutional Review Board Statement: Not applicable.

Informed Consent Statement: Not applicable.

Data Availability Statement: Data are available from the corresponding author upon reasonable request.

Acknowledgments: The staff of the Department of Internal Medicine at the Faculty of Medicine of the University of Debrecen Clinical Center, Hungary are gratefully acknowledged. Ria Benko was supported by The János Bolyai Research Scholarship of the Hungarian Academy of Sciences.

Conflicts of Interest: The authors declare no conflict of interest.

Appendix A

Table A1. Dosage assessment parameters.

Agent	Appropriate (Recommended) Dose			Recommended Dose Adjustment by SPC		Debatable Dose	Underdose/ Overdose
	National CAP Guideline [1]	BTS/NICE CAP Guideline [2]	ATS/IDSA CAP Guideline [2]	eGFR (mL/min)	Body Weight (kg)		
amoxicillin		500 mg orally q8hr or 1g iv[3] q8hr		<10	<50 kg	<50% deviation from the recommended dose and/or absence of loading dose	≥50% deviation from the recommended dose and/or no dose adjustment in renal impairment and in extremes [4] for body weight
amoxicillin-clavulanic acid	500/125 mg or 1/0.25 g q8hr 60/15 mg/kg of body weight/day	500/125mg orally q8hr or 1/0.25g iv[3] q8hr		<10	<50 kg		
clarithromycin	500 mg q12hr	500 mg orally or iv[3] q12hr	500 mg orally or iv[3] q12hr	<30	-		
ceftriaxone	1–2 g iv daily 50–80 mg/kg of body weight		1–2 g iv daily	<30	<40 kg		
moxifloxacin	400 mg daily		400 mg orally or iv[3] daily	<30	-		
levofloxacin	500 mg or 1 g daily	500 mg orally or iv[3] q12hr	750 mg orally or iv[3] daily	≤50	-		
doxycycline		200 mg on first day, then 100 mg daily orally			<50 kg		

CAP—community acquired pneumonia; BTS/NICE—British Thoracic Society/National Institute for Health and Care Excellence; ATS/IDSA—Infectious Diseases Society of America/American Thoracic Society; eGFR—estimated glomerular filtration rate; q8hr—every 8 h; iv—intravenous; q12hr—every 12hours; [1] based on SPC—summary of product characteristics; [2] first-line antibiotic is recommended to give orally when the patient can take oral medicines, and the severity of their condition does not require intravenous antibiotics; antibiotic treatment should be stopped after a total of 5 days unless there is a case of clinical instability; [3] review intravenous antibiotics by 48 h and consider switching to oral antibiotics if possible; [4] extreme body weight: low body weight defined by SPC, and extreme overweight ≥ 100 kg.

References

1. Rossolini, G.M.; Mantengoli, E. Antimicrobial resistance in Europe and its potential impact on empirical therapy. *Clin. Microbiol. Infect.* **2008**, *14* (Suppl. 6), 2–8. [CrossRef] [PubMed]
2. Ghosh, D.; Veeraraghavan, B.; Elangovan, R.; Vivekanandan, P. Antibiotic Resistance and Epigenetics: More to It than Meets the Eye. *Antimicrob. Agents Chemother.* **2020**, *64*, e02225-19. [CrossRef] [PubMed]
3. Antimicrobial Use in European Hospitals. Available online: https://www.ecdc.europa.eu/en/publications-data/antimicrobial-use-european-hospitals (accessed on 19 November 2021).
4. Indication for Antimicrobial Use. Available online: https://www.ecdc.europa.eu/en/healthcare-associated-infections-acute-care-hospitals/database/indications-antimicrobial-use/use (accessed on 12 January 2022).
5. Diagnosis Site of Antimicrobial Treatment. Available online: https://www.ecdc.europa.eu/en/healthcare-associated-infections-acute-care-hospitals/database/indications-antimicrobial-use/diagnosis-site (accessed on 12 January 2022).
6. Respiratory Diseases Statistics. Available online: https://ec.europa.eu/eurostat/statistics-explained/index.php?title=Respiratory_diseases_statistics&oldid=497079#Deaths_from_diseases_of_the_respiratory_system (accessed on 21 January 2022).
7. Brown, J.S. Community-acquired pneumonia. *Clin. Med.* **2012**, *12*, 538–543. [CrossRef]
8. Rider, A.C.; Frazee, B.W. Community-Acquired Pneumonia. *Emerg. Med. Clin. N. Am.* **2018**, *36*, 665–683. [CrossRef]
9. Kaysin, A.; Viera, A.J. Community-Acquired Pneumonia in Adults: Diagnosis and Management. *Am. Fam. Physician* **2016**, *94*, 698–706. [PubMed]
10. OECD; European Union. *Mortality from Respiratory Diseases, in Health at a Glance: Europe 2018: State of Health in the EU Cycle*; OECD Publishing: France, Paris; European Union: Brussels, Belgium, 2018; Available online: https://www.oecd-ilibrary.org/docserver/health_glance_eur-2018-12-en.pdf?expires=1642068861&id=id&accname=guest&checksum=486138DF9F452206CD45EE442FA8CAF1 (accessed on 12 January 2022).
11. Kosar, F.; Alici, D.E.; Hacibedel, B.; Arpinar Yigitbas, B.; Golabi, P.; Cuhadaroglu, C. Burden of community-acquired pneumonia in adults over 18 y of age. *Hum. Vaccin Immunother.* **2017**, *13*, 1673–1680. [CrossRef]

12. Sweeney, J. Panel Finds Widespread Inappropriate Use of Antibiotics in U.S. Hospitals. *Pharm. Today* **2021**, *27*, 52. [CrossRef]
13. Arnold, F.W.; LaJoie, A.S.; Brock, G.N.; Peyrani, P.; Rello, J.; Menendez, R.; Lopardo, G.; Torres, A.; Rossi, P.; Ramirez, J.A.; et al. Improving outcomes in elderly patients with community-acquired pneumonia by adhering to national guidelines: Community-Acquired Pneumonia Organization International cohort study results. *Arch. Intern. Med.* **2009**, *169*, 1515–1524. [CrossRef]
14. Dambrava, P.G.; Torres, A.; Valles, X.; Mensa, J.; Marcos, M.A.; Penarroja, G.; Camps, M.; Estruch, R.; Sanchez, M.; Menendez, R.; et al. Adherence to guidelines' empirical antibiotic recommendations and community-acquired pneumonia outcome. *Eur. Respir. J.* **2008**, *32*, 892–901. [CrossRef]
15. Wathne, J.S.; Harthug, S.; Kleppe, L.K.S.; Blix, H.S.; Nilsen, R.M.; Charani, E.; Smith, I. The association between adherence to national antibiotic guidelines and mortality, readmission and length of stay in hospital inpatients: Results from a Norwegian multicentre, observational cohort study. *Antimicrob. Resist. Infect. Control.* **2019**, *8*, 63. [CrossRef]
16. McCabe, C.; Kirchner, C.; Zhang, H.; Daley, J.; Fisman, D.N. Guideline-concordant therapy and reduced mortality and length of stay in adults with community-acquired pneumonia: Playing by the rules. *Arch. Intern. Med.* **2009**, *169*, 1525–1531. [CrossRef] [PubMed]
17. Frei, C.R.; Restrepo, M.I.; Mortensen, E.M.; Burgess, D.S. Impact of guideline-concordant empiric antibiotic therapy in community-acquired pneumonia. *Am. J. Med.* **2006**, *119*, 865–871. [CrossRef] [PubMed]
18. Matuz, M.; Bognar, J.; Hajdu, E.; Doro, P.; Bor, A.; Viola, R.; Soos, G.; Benko, R. Treatment of Community-Acquired Pneumonia in Adults: Analysis of the National Dispensing Database. *Basic Clin. Pharmacol. Toxicol.* **2015**, *117*, 330–334. [CrossRef] [PubMed]
19. Jackson, C.D.; Burroughs-Ray, D.C.; Summers, N.A. Clinical Guideline Highlights for the Hospitalist: 2019 American Thoracic Society/Infectious Diseases Society of America Update on Community-Acquired Pneumonia. *J. Hosp. Med.* **2020**, *15*, 743–745. [CrossRef] [PubMed]
20. Lim, W.S.; Smith, D.L.; Wise, M.P.; Welham, S.A. British Thoracic Society community acquired pneumonia guideline and the NICE pneumonia guideline: How they fit together. *BMJ Open Respir. Res.* **2015**, *2*, e000091. [CrossRef]
21. Ministry of Health, National Guideline for Antimicrobial Treatment of Community Acquired Pneumonia in Adults with Healthy Immunity, Proffesional Society of Incetious Diseases and Pulmonology. Available online: http://www.tudogyogyasz.hu/upload/tudogyogyasz/document/infektologia_pneumoniak_antimikrobas_kezelese.pdf (accessed on 1 February 2022).
22. National Bacteriological Surveillance Management Team. NBS Annual Reports. National Center for Epidemiology. Available online: www.oek.hu (accessed on 11 December 2021).
23. Silveira, C.D.; Ferreira, C.S.; Correa Rde, A. Adherence to guidelines and its impact on outcomes in patients hospitalized with community-acquired pneumonia at a university hospital. *J. Bras. Pneumol.* **2012**, *38*, 148–157. [CrossRef]
24. Blasi, F.; Iori, I.; Bulfoni, A.; Corrao, S.; Costantino, S.; Legnani, D. Can CAP guideline adherence improve patient outcome in internal medicine departments? *Eur. Respir. J.* **2008**, *32*, 902–910. [CrossRef]
25. Mandell, L.A.; Wunderink, R.G.; Anzueto, A.; Bartlett, J.G.; Campbell, G.D.; Dean, N.C.; Dowell, S.F.; File, T.M., Jr.; Musher, D.M.; Niederman, M.S.; et al. Infectious Diseases Society of America/American Thoracic Society consensus guidelines on the management of community-acquired pneumonia in adults. *Clin. Infect. Dis.* **2007**, *44* (Suppl. 2), S27–S72. [CrossRef]
26. Uranga, A.; Espana, P.P.; Bilbao, A.; Quintana, J.M.; Arriaga, I.; Intxausti, M.; Lobo, J.L.; Tomas, L.; Camino, J.; Nunez, J.; et al. Duration of Antibiotic Treatment in Community-Acquired Pneumonia: A Multicenter Randomized Clinical Trial. *JAMA Intern. Med.* **2016**, *176*, 1257–1265. [CrossRef]
27. Robert, L.; Mark, V.; Moayed, A.; Nivashen, A.; Vinod, R.; Sophie, P.; Mohamed, E.W.; Rusheng, C. Antimicrobial prescribing and outcomes of community-acquired pneumonia in Australian hospitalized patients: A cross-sectional study. *J. Int. Med. Res.* **2021**, *49*, 3000605211058366. [CrossRef]
28. van Heijl, I.; Schweitzer, V.A.; Boel, C.H.E.; Oosterheert, J.J.; Huijts, S.M.; Dorigo-Zetsma, W.; van der Linden, P.D.; Bonten, M.J.M.; van Werkhoven, C.H. Confounding by indication of the safety of de-escalation in community-acquired pneumonia: A simulation study embedded in a prospective cohort. *PLoS ONE* **2019**, *14*, e0218062. [CrossRef] [PubMed]
29. Metlay, J.P.; Waterer, G.W.; Long, A.C.; Anzueto, A.; Brozek, J.; Crothers, K.; Cooley, L.A.; Dean, N.C.; Fine, M.J.; Flanders, S.A.; et al. Diagnosis and Treatment of Adults with Community-acquired Pneumonia. An Official Clinical Practice Guideline of the American Thoracic Society and Infectious Diseases Society of America. *Am. J. Respir. Crit. Care Med.* **2019**, *200*, e45–e67. [CrossRef] [PubMed]
30. Aliberti, S.; Blasi, F.; Zanaboni, A.M.; Peyrani, P.; Tarsia, P.; Gaito, S.; Ramirez, J.A. Duration of antibiotic therapy in hospitalised patients with community-acquired pneumonia. *Eur. Respir. J.* **2010**, *36*, 128–134. [CrossRef] [PubMed]
31. Maxwell, D.J.; McIntosh, K.A.; Pulver, L.K.; Easton, K.L. Empiric management of community-acquired pneumonia in Australian emergency departments. *Med. J. Aust.* **2005**, *183*, 520–524. [CrossRef]
32. Cilli, A.; Sayiner, A.; Celenk, B.; Sakar Coskun, A.; Kilinc, O.; Hazar, A.; Aktas Samur, A.; Tasbakan, S.; Waterer, G.W.; Havlucu, Y.; et al. Antibiotic treatment outcomes in community-acquired pneumonia. *Turk. J. Med. Sci.* **2018**, *48*, 730–736. [CrossRef]
33. Cowling, T.; Farrah, K. *Fluoroquinolones for the Treatment of Respiratory Tract Infections: A Review of Clinical Effectiveness, Cost-Effectiveness, and Guidelines*; Canadian Agency for Drugs and Technologies in Health: Ottawa, ON, Canada, 2019.
34. Liu, S.; Tong, X.; Ma, Y.; Wang, D.; Huang, J.; Zhang, L.; Wu, M.; Wang, L.; Liu, T.; Fan, H. Respiratory Fluoroquinolones Monotherapy vs. beta-Lactams With or Without Macrolides for Hospitalized Community-Acquired Pneumonia Patients: A Meta-Analysis. *Front. Pharmacol.* **2019**, *10*, 489. [CrossRef]

35. Dimopoulos, G.; Matthaiou, D.K.; Karageorgopoulos, D.E.; Grammatikos, A.P.; Athanassa, Z.; Falagas, M.E. Short- versus long-course antibacterial therapy for community-acquired pneumonia: A meta-analysis. *Drugs* **2008**, *68*, 1841–1854. [CrossRef]
36. Zhang, Z.X.; Yong, Y.; Tan, W.C.; Shen, L.; Ng, H.S.; Fong, K.Y. Prognostic factors for mortality due to pneumonia among adults from different age groups in Singapore and mortality predictions based on PSI and CURB-65. *Singap. Med. J.* **2018**, *59*, 190–198. [CrossRef]
37. Conte, H.A.; Chen, Y.T.; Mehal, W.; Scinto, J.D.; Quagliarello, V.J. A prognostic rule for elderly patients admitted with community-acquired pneumonia. *Am. J. Med.* **1999**, *106*, 20–28. [CrossRef]
38. Torres, A.; Peetermans, W.E.; Viegi, G.; Blasi, F. Risk factors for community-acquired pneumonia in adults in Europe: A literature review. *Thorax* **2013**, *68*, 1057–1065. [CrossRef]
39. Torner, N.; Izquierdo, C.; Soldevila, N.; Toledo, D.; Chamorro, J.; Espejo, E.; Fernandez-Sierra, A.; Dominguez, A.; Project, P.I.W.G. Factors associated with 30-day mortality in elderly inpatients with community acquired pneumonia during 2 influenza seasons. *Hum. Vaccin Immunother.* **2017**, *13*, 450–455. [CrossRef] [PubMed]
40. Luna, C.M.; Palma, I.; Niederman, M.S.; Membriani, E.; Giovini, V.; Wiemken, T.L.; Peyrani, P.; Ramirez, J. The Impact of Age and Comorbidities on the Mortality of Patients of Different Age Groups Admitted with Community-acquired Pneumonia. *Ann. Am. Thorac. Soc.* **2016**, *13*, 1519–1526. [CrossRef] [PubMed]
41. Marshall, D.C.; Goodson, R.J.; Xu, Y.; Komorowski, M.; Shalhoub, J.; Maruthappu, M.; Salcicciolo, J.D. Trends in mortality from pneumonia in the Europe union: A temporal analysis of the European detailed mortality database between 2001 and 2014. *Respir. Res.* **2018**, *19*, 81. [CrossRef] [PubMed]
42. Summah, H.; Qu, J.M. Biomarkers: A definite plus in pneumonia. *Mediat. Inflamm.* **2009**, *2009*, 675753. [CrossRef] [PubMed]
43. Ge, Y.L.; Liu, C.H.; Xu, J.; Cui, Z.Y.; Guo, W.C.; Li, H.L.; Fu, A.S.; Wang, H.Y.; Zhang, H.F.; Zhu, X.Y. Serum High-Sensitivity C Reactive Protein Improves Sensitivity of CURB-65 in Predicting ICU Admission and Mortality in Community-Acquired Pneumonia Patients. *Clin. Lab.* **2018**, *64*, 1749–1754. [CrossRef]
44. Almirall, J.; Bolibar, I.; Toran, P.; Pera, G.; Boquet, X.; Balanzo, X.; Sauca, G. Contribution of C-reactive protein to the diagnosis and assessment of severity of community-acquired pneumonia. *Chest* **2004**, *125*, 1335–1342. [CrossRef]
45. Menendez, R.; Martinez, R.; Reyes, S.; Mensa, J.; Polverino, E.; Filella, X.; Esquinas, C.; Martinez, A.; Ramirez, P.; Torres, A. Stability in community-acquired pneumonia: One step forward with markers? *Thorax* **2009**, *64*, 987–992. [CrossRef]
46. Colak, A.; Yilmaz, C.; Toprak, B.; Aktogu, S. Procalcitonin and CRP as Biomarkers in Discrimination of Community-acquired Pneumonia and Exacerbation of COPD. *J. Med. Biochem.* **2017**, *36*, 122–126. [CrossRef]
47. Smith, R.P.; Lipworth, B.J. C-reactive protein in simple community-acquired pneumonia. *Chest* **1995**, *107*, 1028–1031. [CrossRef]
48. Chalmers, J.D.; Singanayagam, A.; Hill, A.T. C-reactive protein is an independent predictor of severity in community-acquired pneumonia. *Am. J. Med.* **2008**, *121*, 219–225. [CrossRef]
49. Andersen, S.; Baunbæk-Knudsen, G.L.; Jensen, A.V.; Petersen, P.T.; Ravn, P. The prognostic value of consecutive C-reactive protein measurements in community acquired pneumonia. *Eur. Respir. J.* **2015**, *46*, 2577.
50. Charlson, M.E.; Pompei, P.; Ales, K.L.; MacKenzie, C.R. A new method of classifying prognostic comorbidity in longitudinal studies: Development and validation. *J. Chronic Dis.* **1987**, *40*, 373–383. [CrossRef]
51. WHO Collaborating Centre for Drug Statistics Methodology, Definition and General Considerations. Available online: https://www.whocc.no/ddd/definition_and_general_considera/ (accessed on 27 January 2022).

MDPI AG
Grosspeteranlage 5
4052 Basel
Switzerland
Tel.: +41 61 683 77 34

Antibiotics Editorial Office
E-mail: antibiotics@mdpi.com
www.mdpi.com/journal/antibiotics

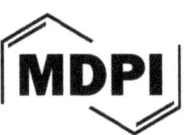

Disclaimer/Publisher's Note: The title and front matter of this reprint are at the discretion of the . The publisher is not responsible for their content or any associated concerns. The statements, opinions and data contained in all individual articles are solely those of the individual Editors and contributors and not of MDPI. MDPI disclaims responsibility for any injury to people or property resulting from any ideas, methods, instructions or products referred to in the content.